Generation
and Interpretation
of the
Electrocardiogram

Generation and Interpretation of the Electrocardiogram

ROBERT PAINE, M.D.

Professor of Clinical Medicine
Washington University Schools of Medicine
St. Louis, Missouri
Chief, Department of Medicine
St. Luke's Hospital
Chesterfield, Missouri

with

Mabel A. Siegel
Lawrence P. Clifford
Daniel M. Dye, M.D.
Chad Magnuson

Lea & Febiger   1988   *Philadelphia*

Lea & Febiger
600 Washington Square
Philadelphia, PA 19106-4198
U.S.A.
(215) 922-1330

Library of Congress Cataloging-in-Publication Data

Paine, Robert, 1921-
   Generation and interpretation of the electrocardiogram.

   Includes index.
   1. Electrocardiography. I. Title.   [DNLM:
1. Electrocardiography.   WG 140 P146g]
RC683.5.E5P28   1988   616.1'207543   87-25996
ISBN 0-8121-1131-1

PRINTED IN THE UNITED STATES OF AMERICA

Print No.   4   3   2   1

To Jane

Whose support, encouragement, and wisdom made this book come to be

Preface

This book has been derived from a series of lectures presented in a senior cardiology elective at St. Luke's Hospital and Washington University Medical School. Over the years, the series has been video recorded for students and house officers. This audience has often requested the additional preparation of a manual for permanent reference.

The book begins with a discussion of the single-cell phenomena from which the electrocardiogram is derived. Subsequent sections discuss the generation of the normal EKG and of the derangements produced by pathologic processes. The basic concepts have been applied to computer generation of electrocardiographic maps of the normal and diseased heart.

In the second half of the book, illustrative electrocardiograms are presented with questions directed to the reader to bring out important points. Data derived from medical records, cardiac catheterization, echocardiography, and nuclear cardiology are correlated. Readers who are familiar with basic electrophysiologic phenomena may prefer to pass over the first and to begin with the second section.

When the questions and answers elicited in the discussion of the electrocardiograms of this section invite further inquiry, the reader may find the desired information by referring to the discussions of basic science in the first section of this book.

We would urge the less advanced reader to "begin at the beginning." It is our hope that this book will help the reader enjoy the application of logic to this reasonable subject. Many of the analogies may appear simplistic, but they are based on solid physiology and anatomy and, as learning aids, have stood the test of time.

Finally, the Appendix presents an original application of computer science, demonstrating the derivation of the electrocardiogram from single-cell events. A few examples of normal and disease states are presented. By modeling, this computer technique allows the prediction of the electrocardiogram in abnormal situations and offers a means of quantitating the disease process involved.

Robert Paine, M.D.

Acknowledgments

In 1964, Carl V. Moore asked us to produce a cardiology elective at St. Luke's Hospital for senior students of Washington University Medical School. This book is, to a considerable degree, derived from the thoughts and inquiries generated by that course. We hereby express our gratitude for Dr. Moore's action and our appreciation to the hundreds of students who have taken this course over the succeeding years. We thank David Kipnis, M.D., for his continued support of this elective in the Department of Internal Medicine of Washington University.

Many others have contributed to the development of this book. St. Luke's Hospital has generously provided space, personnel, and other resources. Especially, Audrey Richardson and the St. Luke's Heart Station have labored faithfully to provide illustrative electrocardiograms. Deborah Hobbs-Murphy, St. Luke's Medical Librarian, has provided essential assistance on many occasions. The St. Luke's Medical Records Department has produced essential data for clinical correlation. Linda Anderson has guided us in the preparation of the manuscript for critical review.

Our thanks also go to Peter Corr, M.D., of the Department of Pharmacology of Washington University.

To Daniel M. Dye, M.D., belongs the credit for recognizing the potential use of the computer in relating single-cell phenomena to whole-heart electrical recordings.

Especially to Chad Magnuson we express our thanks for the painstaking and exquisitely accurate computer studies.

To Lawrence P. Clifford we owe appreciation for the illustrations and photographs without which this book would be of little value.

Contents

PART I

Generation of the Electrocardiogram

SINGLE-CELL ELECTROPHYSIOLOGY

A working contractile myocardial cell at end diastole is represented in Figure I–1. The chief cation within the cell is $K^+ \bullet^+$: the most numerous extracellular cation is $Na^+ \bullet^+$; the chief extracellular anion is $Cl^- \circ$. Considerable emphasis should be placed on the predominant intracellular anion, the negatively charged protein molecule too large to diffuse through the sarcolemma. Let us consider the behavior of the K (potassium) ions highly concentrated in the cytoplasm (140 mEq/L). They will diffuse outward down their concentration gradient until the resulting spatial separation of cation-anion pairs (K-protein) generates an electrical gradient (the resting potential) equal and opposite to the concentration gradient. A cartoonist might represent the resting situation as a halo of K^+ ions surrounding the cell, with its negative protein inside. The normal 90-mV resting potential recorded by intra- and extracellular electrodes is shown in Figure I–2.

Let us alter one portion of the sarcolemma, as one might open a venetian blind, and allow the Na (sodium) ions to pass rapidly through under the impetus of both their concentration gradient and the electrical gradient (Figure I–3). The rapid invasion of Na through rapid sarcolemmal channels into the negatively charged cytoplasm creates an almost instantaneous elimination of the trans-sarcolemmal potential and is represented by the rapid upstroke of the action potential recorded by an intracellular probe (Figure I–2). This initial upstroke (phase 0) thus represents Na^+ entry (Figure I–4). The migration of positive Na ions into the cytoplasm permits further escape of K (Figure I–5, phase

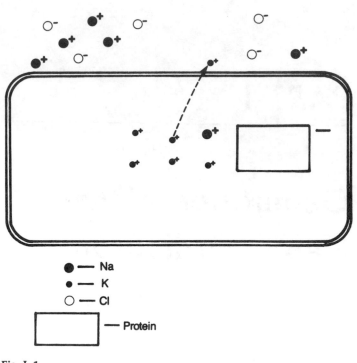

$\bullet$ — Na
$\bullet$ — K
$\circ$ — Cl

— Protein

Fig. I–1

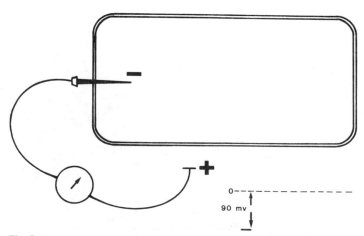

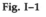

0 – – – – – – – – – – – –
90 mv

Fig. I–2

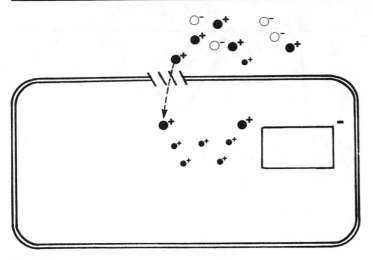

Fig. I–3

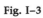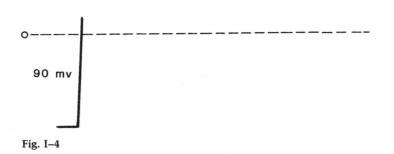

90 mv

Fig. I–4

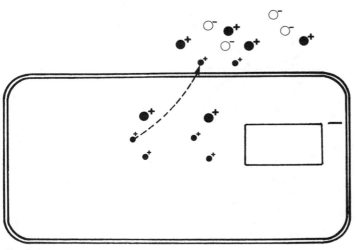

Fig. I–5

3) until once again K concentration gradient and the electrical gradient are balanced. Thus, Na entry is followed by potassium exit, which restores the resting potential (Figure I–6). Between the rapid entry of Na (phase 0) and exit of K (phase 3), the positive spike (phase 1, possibly the result of chloride escape) and the plateau (phase 2) occur. During phase 2, Ca (calcium) enters through slow sarcolemmal channels (Figure I–7). Contractile myocardial cells maintain resting potential during diastole (phase 4) (Figure I–8).

To this point, ionic movement has been down concentration gradients, requiring no cellular work (like apples falling from trees). If each beat were associated only with Na entry and K escape, cells would rapidly become sodium-laden and potassium-deficient and would cease functioning. Na/K ATPase in the sarcolemma energizes the expulsion of sodium and the retrieval of potassium by the cells, especially during the latter portion of the action potential (Figure I–9). Thus, ions are placed "back on the shelf" by the completion of each action potential.

Let us consider the process of conduction (Figure I–10). Because we have likened the sarcolemma to a venetian blind for Na entry, let us carry the simple analogy a bit further and observe the *possible* behavior of Na⁺ ions "downstream" from the "open" segment. Lateral migration of Na to the "open" segment might reduce the transmembrane potential in that segment from which Na moved and, in an unexplained manner, trigger the opening of another section of venetian blind. Alternatively, conduction might be likened to "opening" the sarcolemma in a "domino effect." In either case, the speed of entry of Na⁺ in phase 0 is directly correlated with the speed of conduction (Figure I–11). We will see later that drugs that delay Na entry predictably slow conduction.

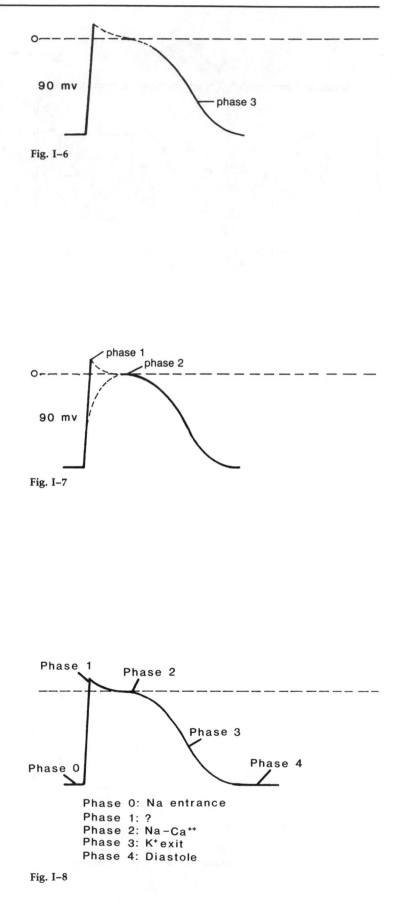

Fig. I–6

Fig. I–7

Phase 0: Na entrance
Phase 1: ?
Phase 2: Na–Ca⁺⁺
Phase 3: K⁺ exit
Phase 4: Diastole

Fig. I–8

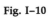
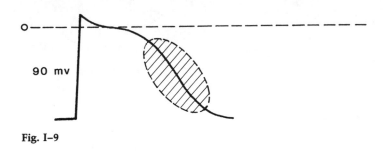

Fig. I–9

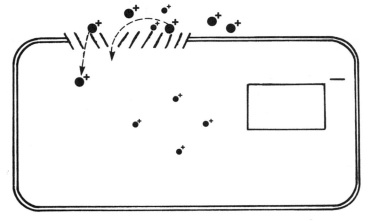

Fig. I–10

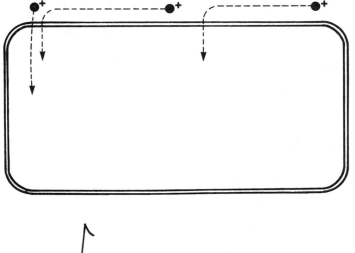

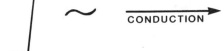
CONDUCTION

Fig. I–11

RELATION OF SINGLE-CELL TO WHOLE-HEART ELECTRICAL PHENOMENA

To this point, we have considered *trans-sarcolemmal* single-cell events. As we shall see, the electrocardiogram is generated by the *surface* charges on the myriad of cells that comprise the myocardium. The ventricular myocardium is shown schematically in Figure I–12. Note the thin apex and thick base of the left ventricle and the thin free wall of the right ventricle, because these anatomic features are important in the production of the ventricular electrocardiogram. In Figure I–13, the A-V node, the common bundle of His and the intraventricular conducting system are diagrammed. The Purkinje fibers first penetrate the septal myocardium near the cardiac apex and thereafter are distributed in the subendocardium from the apex to the equator of the ventricles.

The absence of specialized conduction apparatus in the basal half of the ventricles and the near-apical site of initial stimulation of the ventricles appears to ensure against outflow obstruction by premature contraction of the basal circular muscles. Figure I–14 demonstrates the initial "beach head" of depolarization produced by Na^+ invasion of cells. A magnified diagram of this colony of cells (Figure I–15) illustrates the fundamental process generating the biologic battery (dipole), from which the electrocardiogram is derived. The subendocardial tier of cells has been invaded by Na^+, causing a loss of positive charge on the surface. In Figure I–16, depolarization has advanced further into the adjoining rank of cells. It is essential to recognize that inequality of surface charges produces the dipole as it progresses across the

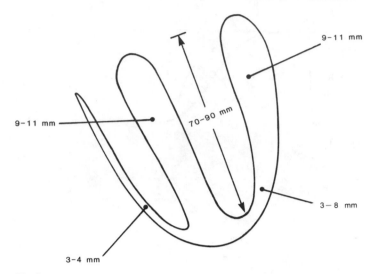

Fig. I–12

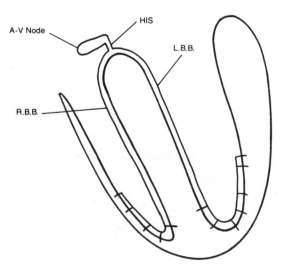

Fig. I–13

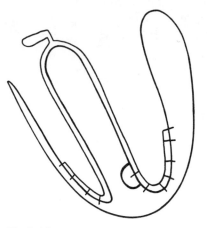

Fig. I–14

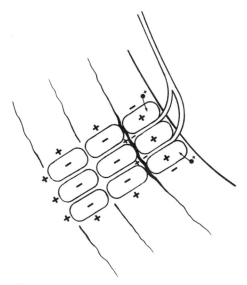

Fig. I–15

Comments/Group

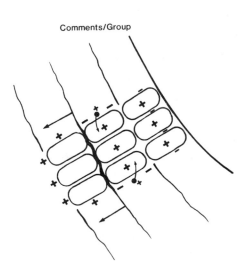

Fig. I–16

myocardium (rather like a threshing machine advancing across a "positive" standing wheat field, leaving in its trail the "negative" horizontal stalks). The interface of positive and negative surface charges generates the electrical field seen in Figure I–17. Examine the behavior of a single electron in Figure I–17: it is repelled by the negative pole of the dipole and attracted by the positive; and, free to move in the body, it follows the pathway as shown. Its sister electrons, also free to move in the volume conductor of the body, swing in similar orbits, the most superficial of these arching to the skin as seen in Figure I–18.

If we were to build a crude EKG machine in our basement workshop, we would need a metal plate to apply to the skin and alcohol or a similar substance to reduce the resistance to the passage of the free electron (Figure I–18) from the body into our machine. We would use a low-resistance wire to connect our metal electrode to an infinite capacitor (earth) (Figure I–19). Thus, our machine is in fact an electron trap, offering less than body resistance to the flow of electrons set in motion by the dipole. The final requirement of our homemade machine would be some mechanism to measure the electron traffic along our wire. For this, we use a horseshoe magnet and we suspend our wire between its poles, running at 90° to the plane of the magnet (Figure I–20). The suspended wire serves as the stylus of our machine, moving toward the North Pole when electron traffic moves one way and to the South Pole when traffic is in reverse. [This behavior no doubt will recall the subject of motors and generators in high school physics.] Clinical EKG machines differ from our model in their filters and amplifiers and elaborate styluses but not in their fundamental principles. By

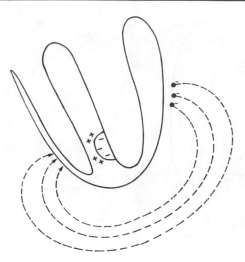

Fig. I–17

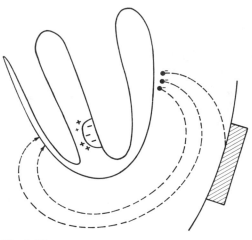

Fig. I–18

Comments/Group

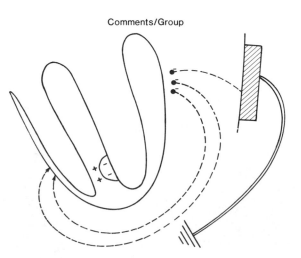

Fig. I–19

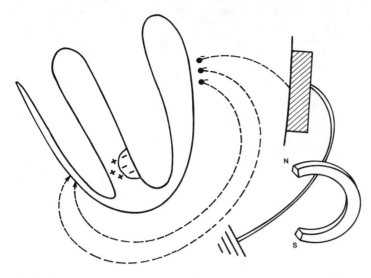

Fig. I–20

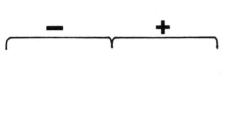

Fig. I–21

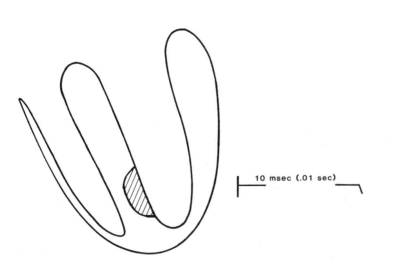

Fig. I–22

mutual consent, all manufacturers design their EKG machines to record a downward deflection when the electrode faces the negative aspect of the dipole and electrons are donated from the patient to the machine; when the electrode faces the positive pole of the dipole, electrons are donated from the machine to the patient and an upright deflection is recorded. Figure I–21 re-emphasizes the fact that it is the surface charges on the cells that produce the dipole.

Depolarization of the ventricles is initiated on the left side of the septum near the apex; 10 msec into the depolarization process, the dipole lies as shown in Figure I–22. Invasion of septal cells by Na thereafter advances as shown in Figures I–23 and I–24, generating an initially negative (Q-wave) deflection in left-sided leads (Figures I–22, I–23, I–24). By 20 msec, septal depolarization is complete.

At 30 msec, the dipole front has moved down the bundle branches and into the penetrating filaments (Figure I–25). As seen in Figure I–26, these terminal Purkinje twigs penetrate a few millimeters into the myocardium and induce depolarization of the surrounding cells. These colonies of Na-invaded cells are of special importance because their spherical shape produces self-cancellation of dipoles (Figure I–27). Thus, the subendocardial-myocardial depolarization produces no net dipole. As we shall see, subendocardial infarction produces no pathologic Q wave, because loss of this tissue produces no dipole loss.

By 40 msec, the subendocardial depolarization shown in Figures I–26 and I–27 has expanded so that opposing or cancelling wave fronts no longer exist and the situation seen in Figure I–28 is present. Thus, by 40 msec, left-sided electrodes record upright deflections (R waves). This is such a consistent

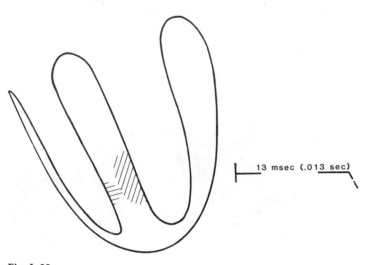

13 msec (.013 sec)

Fig. I–23

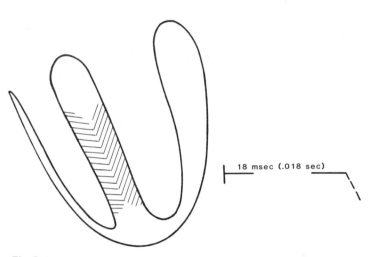

18 msec (.018 sec)

Fig. I–24

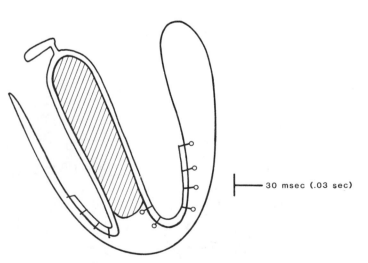

30 msec (.03 sec)

Fig. I–25

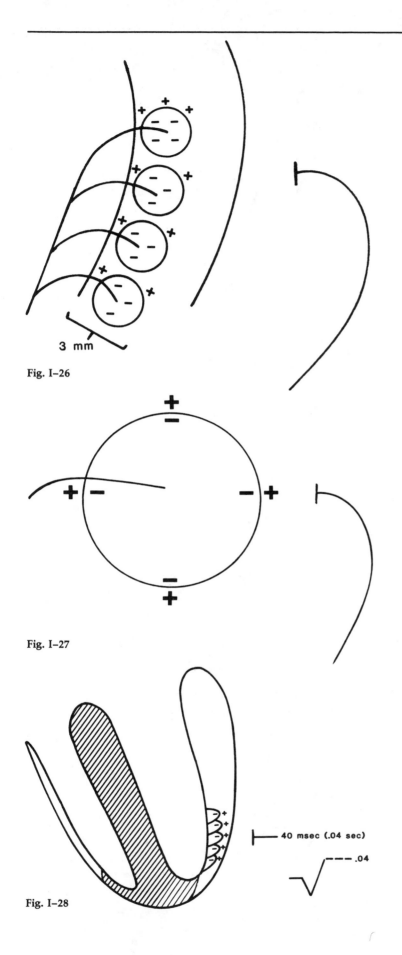

Fig. I–26

Fig. I–27

Fig. I–28

40 msec (.04 sec)

----- .04

phenomenon in normal humans, EKG paper is divided in .04-sec (40-msec) units to facilitate recognition of pathologic .04-sec Q waves.

Because the Purkinje network extends only part way up the free walls of the left and right ventricles, the later stages of free-wall depolarization occur as shown in Figures I–29 through I–32.

Note the effect of the change in electrode position shown in Figures I–33 and I–34. As the dipole moves past the electrode, its negative pole faces the electrode and produces an S wave.

The normal time required for ventricular depolarization is .05 to .08 sec. This represents the elapsed time from the first depolarization of cells on the left side of the septum to depolarization of the last cells to be invaded by Na^+ at the base of the left ventricular free wall.

The normal ventricular depolarization thus begins on the left side of the septum and advances in a cranial and caudal direction. Depolarization begins on the right side of the septum shortly after the beachhead is established on the left. We will see later that normal variation of the location of these beachheads can produce clinically important consequences. By 20 msec, the septal process is complete. The dipole front advancing toward the apex produces the 30-msec portion of the QRS complex; the spherical areas of depolarization in the inner 3 mm of the free wall of the left ventricle self-cancel and make no contribution to QRS generation. From 40 sec on, the array of dipoles advancing outward and headward through the free left ventricular wall generates the remaining portion of the QRS.

Thus, an electrode placed to the left of the normal heart records an initially negative septal Q wave. The deflection at 30 msec is

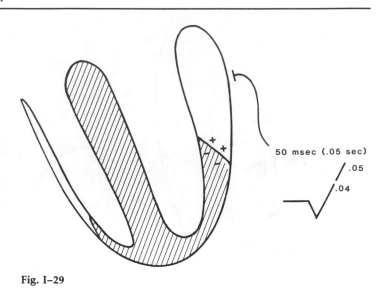

Fig. I–29

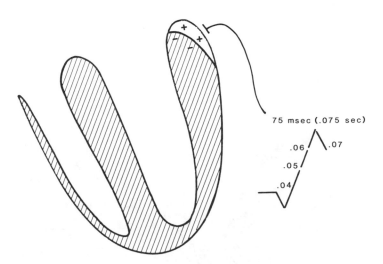

Fig. I–30

Fig. I–31

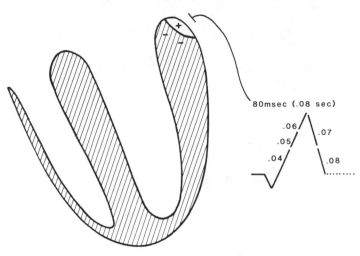

80msec (.08 sec)

Fig. I–32

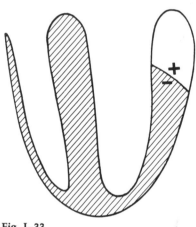

Dipole passing directly across
axis of electrode records equality of
+ and −, and stylus returns to baseline

Fig. I–33

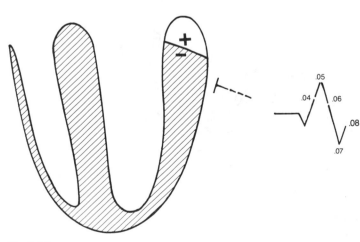

Fig. I–34

positive or negative, depending on the position of the electrode relative to the dipole advancing toward the apex. In all normal humans, the left-sided electrode records an upright R wave before 40 msec. The terminal portion of the QRS is normally positive or negative, depending on the position of the electrode relative to the dipoles advancing through the basal free wall. It should be mentioned that depolarization of the free wall of the right ventricle normally is obscured by the dipoles generated in the more massive left ventricle. Indeed, the *normal* right ventricle can be surgically extirpated without affecting the *normal* EKG.

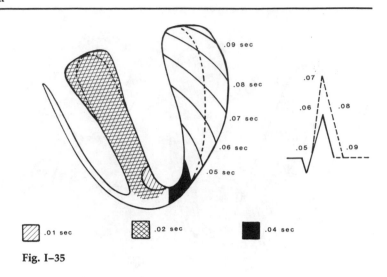

Fig. I–35

LEFT VENTRICULAR HYPERTROPHY

Let us now examine the changes in QRS produced by hypertrophy of the left ventricle. As shown in Figure I–35, the initial septal events are normal, whereas the dipole fronts at .05 to .08 sec are broader than normal, and depolarization of the base is not completed within the normal time. A left-sided electrode would register a taller R wave than normal, and QRS duration would be longer than normal. The normal septal Q wave would be preserved. A right-sided electrode would record a normal initial R wave from septal depolarization and an abnormally large S wave. The terminal wave recorded from the left would be positive (R) or negative (S), depending on the relation of the electrodes to the terminal basal dipoles.

LEFT BUNDLE BRANCH BLOCK

When the left bundle is interrupted (left bundle branch block) as illustrated in Figure

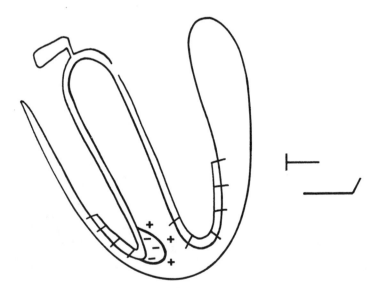

Fig. I–36

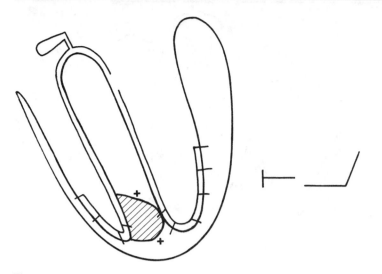

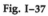

Fig. I–37

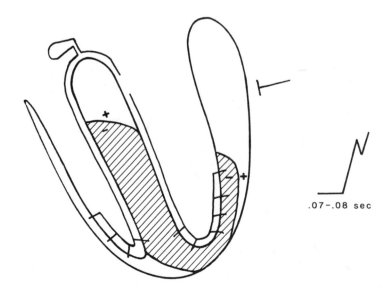

.07–.08 sec

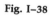

Fig. I–38

I–36, with survival of its lower components (analogous to a highway with a bridge washed out), entry into the ventricles is via the right bundle and initial depolarization is on the right side of the septum. Septal dipoles move toward the left, as shown in Figures I–36 and I–37. Left-sided electrodes register an initial R wave, distinguishing this situation from normal and from left-ventricular hypertrophy. As the dipole wave reaches the surviving radicals of the left bundle system, depolarization is conducted in normal sequence to the free wall of the left ventricle Figs. I–38 through I–40). Figure I–41 may be helpful in visualizing the process of depolarization. One might imagine the heart made of bricks, each surrounded by a positive coat of mortar. As Na^+ invasion occurs, the positive mortar becomes negative. The dipole is generated by the close approximation of positive mortar and negative mortar. The strength of the dipole at any moment is determined in part by the number of bricks involved at the interface between positive and negative mortar. Depolarization of the narrow isthmus at the apex of the left ventricle produces a weaker (and downward-directed) dipole than the broader dipole advancing through the free wall. As a result, a notch may occur on the QRS.

A second form of left bundle block is shown in Figure I–42. Here, the interruption of the proximal left bundle is accompanied by cessation of conduction down the lower reaches of the left bundle system. This is analogous to the death of a peripheral nerve when a proximal lesion exists. Thus, we could call this the "cut nerve" form of left bundle branch block. Initial septal depolarization is by way of the right bundle, and left-sided leads register an initial R wave.

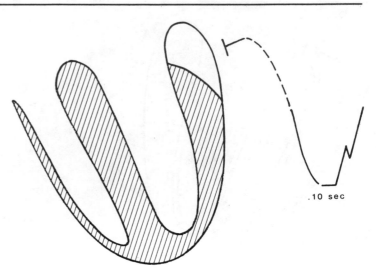

Fig. I–39

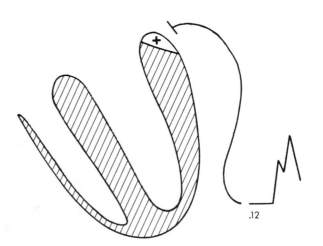

Fig. I–40

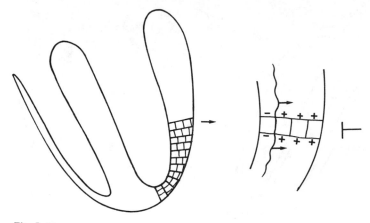

Fig. I–41

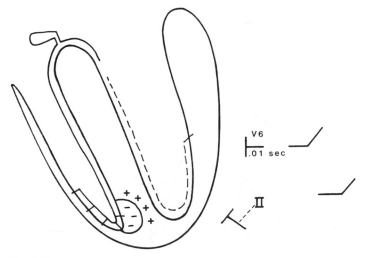

Fig. I–42

When the dipole front reaches the left side of the septum, no left bundle apparatus is functioning. Advance of the dipoles is, therefore, by way of the contractile myocardium (Figs. I–43 through I–48). The apex-to-base direction of free-wall depolarization causes caudal electrodes (II, III, aVF) to be in the negative field generated by free-wall dipoles. Large terminal S waves are registered in these leads, producing left axis deviation (see later discussion). The long path from apex to base significantly prolongs the time required for ventricular depolarization. This form of LBBB is distinguished by (1) left axis deviation, (2) large terminal S waves (in leads II, III, aVF, and V₃), and (3) markedly prolonged QRS (.14 sec or longer). The "washed-out bridge" LBBB as a solitary lesion most frequently prolongs the QRS to .12 sec. As one might expect, the first form of LBBB might be produced by focal disease, often ischemic; whereas the second form most often results from diffuse myocardiomyopathy or multiple foci of ischemic damage.

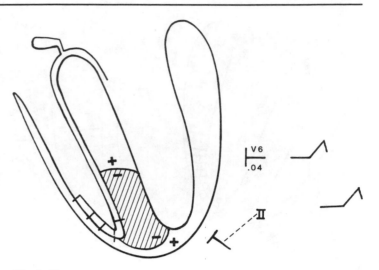

Fig. I–43

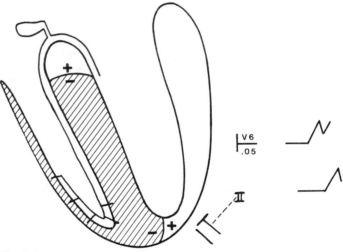

Fig. I–44

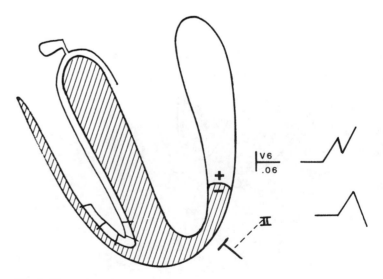

Fig. I–45

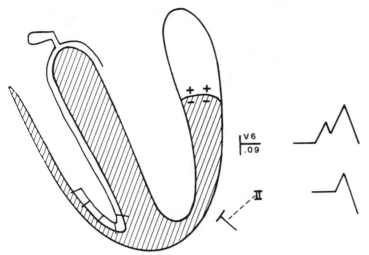

Fig. I-46

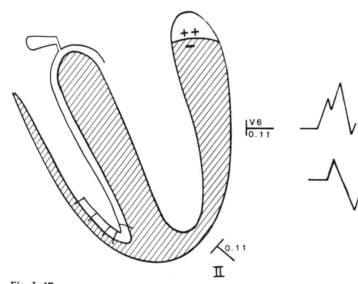

Fig. I-47

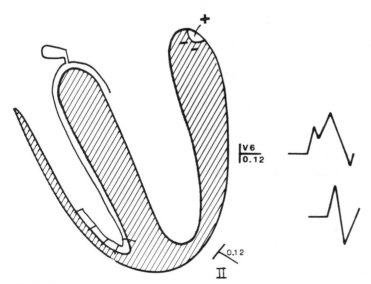

Fig. I-48

RIGHT BUNDLE BRANCH BLOCK

Right bundle branch block (RBBB) (Figs. I–49 through I–55) does not alter depolarization of the left septum, the apex, or the free wall of the left ventricle. The septal Q wave is not prolonged despite the loss of right septal depolarization, because left ventricular free-wall dipoles are formed on time (Fig. I–51), and their positive poles facing leftward terminate the left negative field generated by septal dipoles. Thus, as we shall see, RBBB does not produce false evidence of myocardial infarction. The hallmarks of RBBB are produced by the late invasion of the free wall of the right ventricle. Although this wall is only 3- to 4-mm thick, the march of dipoles is not from endo- to epicardium in RBBB, but is from apex to base, normally a length of 70 to 90 mm. The dipoles are oriented with positive poles to the right anteriorly and superiorly and negative poles to the left and inferiorly. Thus, the terminal wave in right-sided leads is positive (R') and in left-sided leads is negative (S). Thus V_1 registers RsR' and V_6 registers qRs.

It is the long (70- to 90-mm) course of free-wall depolarization that generates the prolongation of QRS duration. It is customary to classify right and left bundle branch block as incomplete when QRS duration is less than .12 sec. Although this is common practice, it is important to recognize that the time from initial septal invasion to final basal depolarization (QRS duration) in both RBBB and LBBB is influenced by the speed of intramyocardial conduction and by the size of the heart. Thus, a midget with bundle branch block might have a QRS of .10 or so, whereas the QRS of a giant with bundle block might measure, .15 sec or so. This does not deny the existence of incomplete bundle block, but

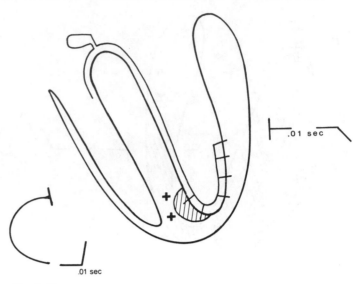

Fig. I–49

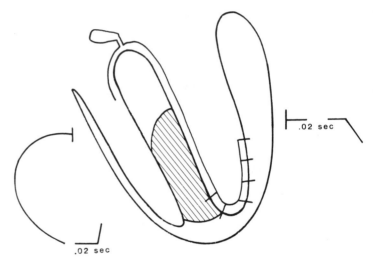

Fig. I–50

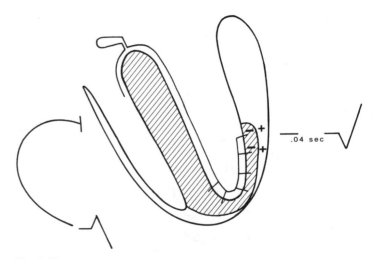

Fig. I–51

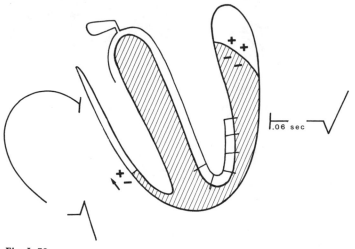

Fig. I–52

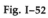

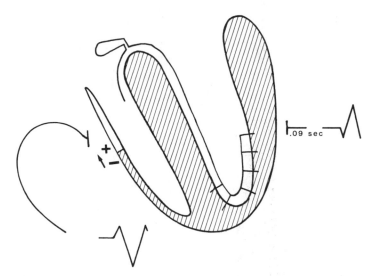

Fig. I–53

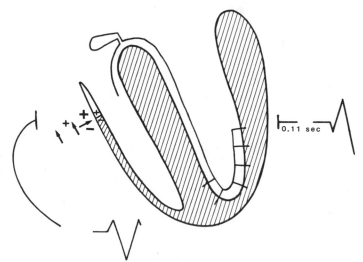

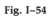

Fig. I–54

rather points out the fact that .12 sec is not necessarily a diagnostic number.

A common variant may result from a foreshortened or bobtailed right bundle (Figs. I–56 and I–57). In such individuals, prolongation of depolarization up the free wall of the right ventricle produces some lengthening of the QRS and RsR′ in V_1 and qRs in V_6. This delay may add .02 sec to the QRS. Thus, an otherwise normal individual with the harmless abnormality of the right bundle may have normal or slightly prolonged QRS duration, depending on the QRS he would have had without the shortened bundle. This variant in an otherwise normal individual is of no consequence and has no effect on life expectancy.

In the presence of right ventricular dilatation with extension of the free wall of the right ventricle, a similar prolongation of QRS with late R′ in right-sided leads and S in left leads occurs. One may not be able to distinguish between right ventricular dilatation and RBBB (Fig. I–58).

REPOLARIZATION: THE T WAVE

The T wave is the product of phase 3 repolarization of the ventricular myocardial cells. During this phase, the positive external charge around the sarcolemma is restored by K escape and Na extrusion, and the cytoplasmic charge becomes negative once again (Fig. I–59).

The septal apical region repolarizes first for two reasons: (1) These cells are the first to be invaded by Na$^+$ (depolarized); therefore, they are the first to reach phase 3 (repolarization). (2) The apical wall is thin, therefore apical myocardial layers depolarize and repolarize earlier than thicker layers of the remainder of the ventricles (Fig. I–60).

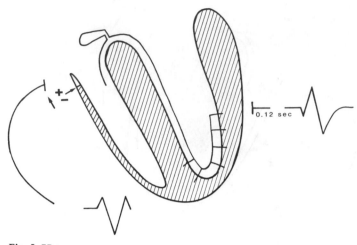

Fig. I–55

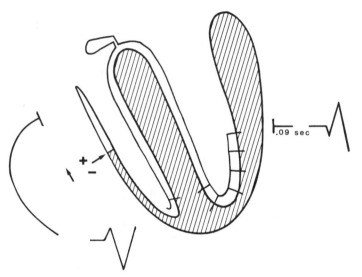

Fig. I–56

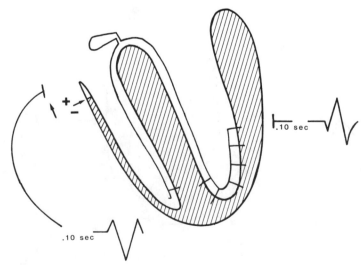

Fig. I–57

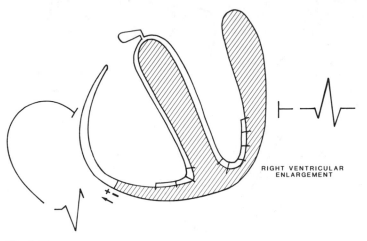

RIGHT VENTRICULAR
ENLARGEMENT

Fig. I–58

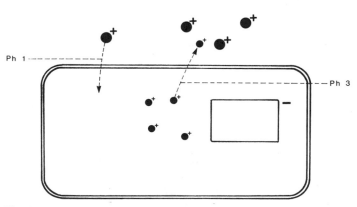

Ph 1

Ph 3

Fig. I–59

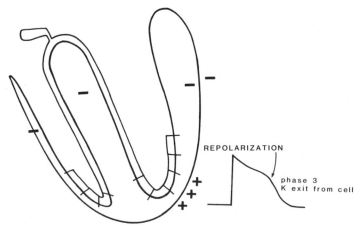

REPOLARIZATION

phase 3
K exit from cell

Fig. I–60

Therefore, repolarization advances from apex to base (Figs. I–61, I–62, I–63).

The duration of the action potential of myocardial cells decreases from endocardium to epicardium. As a result, more superficial myocardial cells recover positive surface charge (repolarize) earlier than deeper cells, even though they were depolarized later. Important participants in this phenomenon are the Purkinje network in the subendocardium. One might *speculate* about the mechanism of the prolonged action potentials of these cells when compared with the remainder of the myocardial cellular population. One factor might be considered the presence of transverse canals across the contractile cells (Fig. I–64). These invaginations through the sarcolemma probably serve to facilitate Na^+ and Ca^+ entry into the milieu of the contractile apparatus within the cytoplasm. They may also act as conduits facilitating K^+ exit during phase 3 (Fig. I–65).

Without transverse canals, Purkinje cells might be expected to repolarize more slowly than the contractile population. If one wished to speculate further, one could relate the tenfold increase in conduction velocity of the Purkinje cells to the absence of detours through transverse canal byways. We should emphasize the purely conjectural nature of the proposal.

Whether or not these simple concepts are valid, Purkinje cells conduct much more rapidly and repolarize much more slowly than do contractile cells; and more superficial cells repolarize before deeper cells. These anatomic and physiologic factors ensure the repolarization of the more superficial layers of the myocardium before the subendocardium and the apical before the more basal myocardium (Fig. I–66).

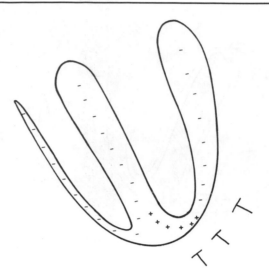

Fig. I–61

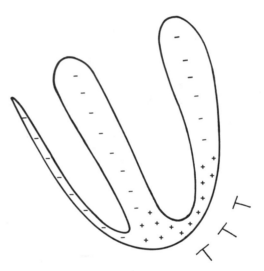

Fig. I–62

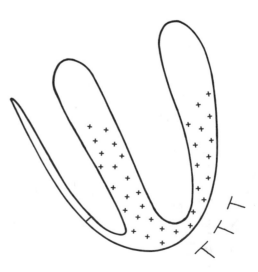

Fig. I–63

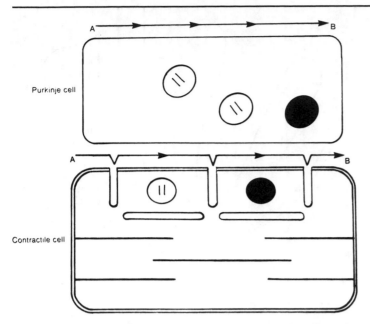

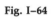

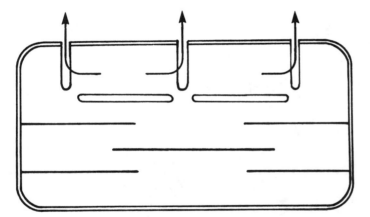

PURKINJE A to B 10x CONTRACTILE CELL

Fig. I–64

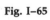

Fig. I–65

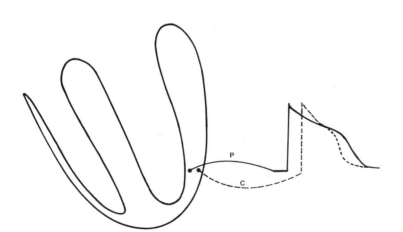

Fig. I–66

The action potentials of two cells super-imposed in proper time sequence are shown in Figures I–66 and I–67. The differences between simultaneous surface charges are indicated by the vertical lines of Figure I–67. During depolarization, Na invasion of the subendocardial cell is more advanced than the simultaneous invasion of the superficial contractile cell. At each moment during phase 0, the surface charge of the superficial cell is more positive than the subendocardial cell. The resultant dipole produces an upright (R wave) deflection on the surface lead positioned as shown in Figure I–67. During phase 2, the cells are equally depolarized and the resultant S-T segment is isoelectric. In phase 3, the prolonged action potential of the subendocardial cell produces a dipole that derives its shape from the S shape of phase 3. The EKG of the two-cell model has a sharp QRS because it is derived from the abrupt upstroke of phase 0; whereas the T wave is a rolling hummock because of its derivation from the curvature of phase 3.

We have accounted for the positivity of the T wave in apical leads. We must also explain the normal positivity of anterior and left lateral leads. To do so, it is important to remember the shape of the ventricles. The mass of the left ventricle facing anteriorly and laterally far exceeds the mass facing rightward and posteriorly, because the orifices of the atrioventricular and semilunar valves replace a significant segment of wall. We are recording the EKG of a horseshoe rather than a sphere (Fig. I–68). If this were not so, the EKG would be a flat line because the dipoles of equal and opposite walls would cancel. The special contribution of the septum to the magnification of anterior and lateral dipoles will be discussed later.

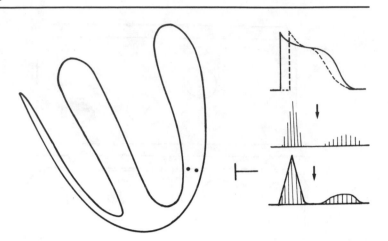

Fig. I–67

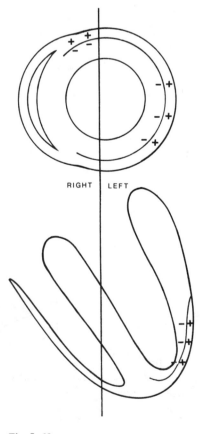

Fig. I–68

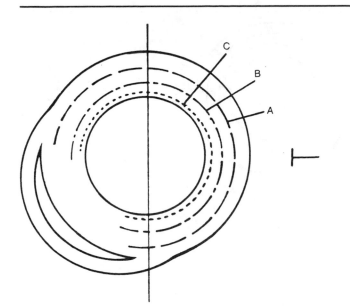

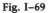
Fig. I-69

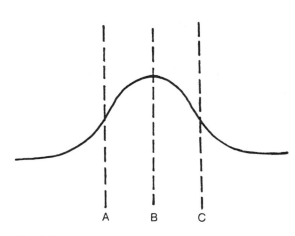

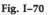
Fig. I-70

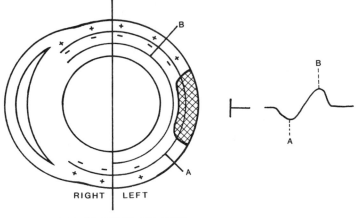

RIGHT | LEFT

LOSS OF CELLS ON LEFT

Fig. I-71

Although depolarization advances from inside out and repolarization from outside in, it is helpful to recognize that, whereas depolarization advances in rapid sequence across the septum, centrifugally through the apex and the free wall, and finally upward along the basal free wall of the left ventricle, repolarization advances from the epicardial apex toward the endocardium and base of the ventricles.

It may be useful to illustrate this process with numbers. Let us suppose that an electrode faces 1 million positive dipoles in the adjacent wall in ring A (Fig. I-69) and .5 million negative dipoles in the opposite wall. Thus, the proximal wall outnumbers the far wall by .5 million units. The lead at this moment would register a .5-million-unit positive deflection. At time B, the proximal dipoles might number 1.5 million and the opposite wall .75 million, and the recorded deflection would increase to .75 units. At ring C, with a diminishing number of dipoles (as the depolarized population shrinks), the adjacent population may number .75 million and the opposite .375 million, and the lead would register .375 units. The normal T wave would appear as seen in Figure I-70. The early portion of the T wave is an apical, subepicardial event, the mid-portion, a mid-wall event, and the final portion is subendocardial, basal in origin.

Bearing this in mind, we can anticipate the T-wave abnormality generated by lesions in various locations. If, as shown in Figure I-71, the outer stratum of the adjacent wall has been destroyed, the T wave will register the loss of positive dipoles facing the lead, and if the number of opposite-wall negative poles facing the electrode exceeds the number of proximal-wall positive poles, the initial T wave is negative. If, instead, the middle layer is destroyed, the mid-portion of the T wave is inverted; if the subendocardial myocardium is electrically inert, the terminal T wave is inverted (Fig. I–72). If there is a transmural loss, the T is inverted and, taking its shape from the phenomenon illustrated in Figure I–70, is *symmetrically* inverted (Fig. I–73). We will return to this important point later. If the opposite wall has been destroyed, the positive charge of the adjacent dipoles is magnified, and tall symmetrical T waves are seen in the overlying lead.

We have considered the effects on T waves of the loss of cells; the same phenomenon would occur if pathologic change caused a prolongation of the action potential, because in the "race" against the opposite wall, the delayed adjacent wall would "lose" and the T would invert. Likewise, a delay in conduction to the adjacent wall would cause the adjacent wall to lose the repolarization race with the opposite wall (Fig. I–74).

If the plateau of phase 2 is not horizontal, but is increasingly on a downslope as it approaches phase 3, the difference in simultaneous surface charge would increase from QRS to T wave, with the delayed wall increasingly delayed in the generation of positive dipole when compared with the opposite normal wall (Fig. I–75). If, however, phase 2 is isoelectric, with no downward tilt, delay can produce a symmetrically inverted T wave.

THE S-T SEGMENT AND SEVERE INJURY

Let us consider other *diastolic* events. Normally, the myocardial cell resembles a boat with a built-in leakiness of the hull (sarcolemma) compensated for by a built-in bailer

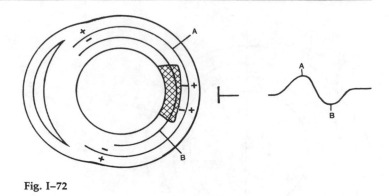

Fig. I–72

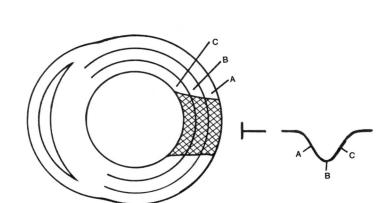

Fig. I–73

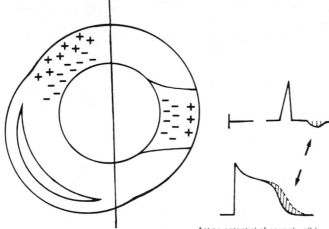

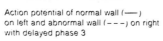

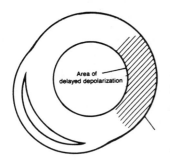

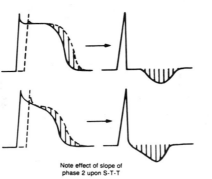

Action potential of normal wall (——)
on left and abnormal wall (– – –) on right
with delayed phase 3

Fig. I–74

Area of
delayed depolarization

Note effect of slope of
phase 2 upon S-T-T

Fig. I–75

(the sarcolemmal Na-K ATPase). The bailer is energized by oxidation. As a result, the bottom of the "boat" stays almost "dry." The depth of the bottom of the boat below the water line is comparable to the normal resting potential (Fig. I–76). When the sarcolemma is damaged, it may be more leaky or its Na-K ATPase may falter in its bailing function. As a result, more salt water collects in the boat-cell. As salt water accumulates in the boat-cell, the resting potential decreases (Fig. I–77).

Consider the consequences of damage to a colony of myocardial cells (Fig. I–78). Because of sarcolemmal leaking or of sarcolemmal pump dysfunction, these cells contain increased amounts of sodium and water and their resting potentials are less than 90 mV. A lead placed over this colony (Fig. I–79) would register the presence of a dipole between the normal cells and the injured cells.

If the resting potential of the injured cell were 60 mV, this 60–90 *diastolic dipole* will depress the *diastolic baseline* 30 mV (Fig. I–79). With initiation of septal depolarization, an additional negative deflection will occur (Fig. I–80). The sequential depolarization of the ventricles will produce the positive R wave (Figs. I–81, I–82, and I–83), until finally,

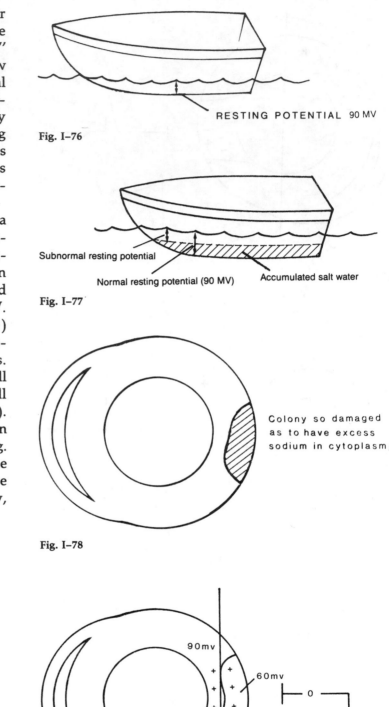

Fig. I–76

RESTING POTENTIAL 90 MV

Subnormal resting potential

Normal resting potential (90 MV)   Accumulated salt water

Fig. I–77

Colony so damaged as to have excess sodium in cytoplasm

Fig. I–78

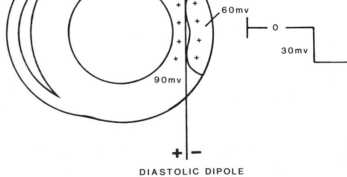

90mv

60mv

0

30mv

90mv

DIASTOLIC DIPOLE

Fig. I–79

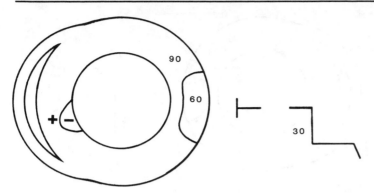

Fig. I–80

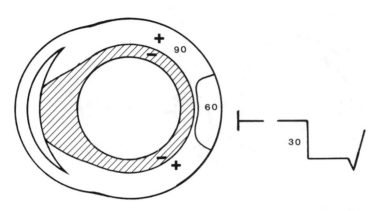

Fig. I–81

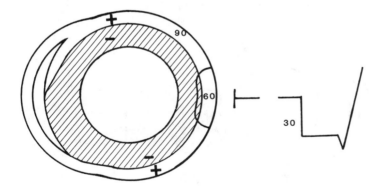

Fig. I–82

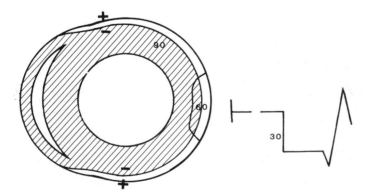

Fig. I–83

when all ventricular cells have been depolarized (Fig. I–84), the stylus returns to true zero. Repolarization (Fig. I–85) reestablishes the abnormality of surface charges of the damaged colony, and the stylus returns to the false baseline (−30 mV) (Figs. I–86, I–87, I–88).

Because EKG machines are built with a stylus adjustment that provides for selection of position of the tracing on the paper, we have no way of knowing the location of true zero and we see an illusory S-T elevation, when in fact, there is a baseline depression (Fig. I–89).

If the colony of severely damaged cells lies in the subendocardial layers of the adjacent wall, the diastolic dipole 90–60 will produce a 30-mV baseline elevation (Fig. I–90). Systolic depolarization thereafter generates a

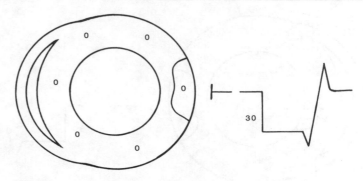

Fig. I–84

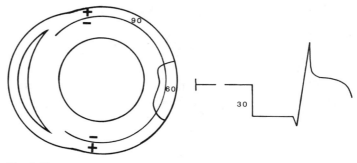

Fig. I–85

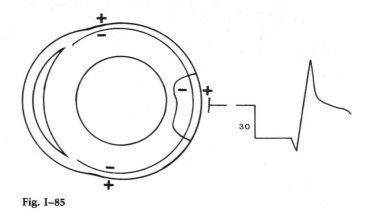

Fig. I–86

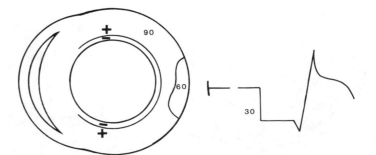

Fig. I–87

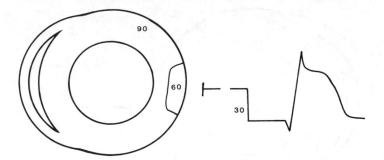

Fig. I–88

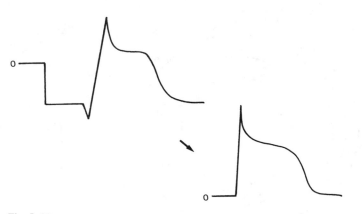

Fig. I–89

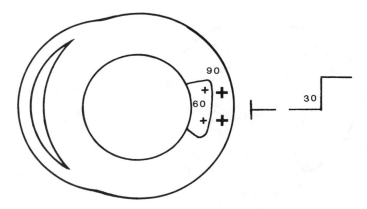

Fig. I–90

septal Q and free-wall R wave (Figs. I–91, I–92, and I–93). When all cells are equally depolarized, the stylus returns to true zero, 30 mV below the apparent baseline (Fig. I–94). Once again, repolarization reestablishes an inequality of charges and the stylus inscribes a phase-3-like return to the baseline. Thus, not knowing the location of true zero, we see the illusion of S-T depression.

If severe transmural damage occurs to the adjacent wall, an electrode placed directly over the lesion responds to the 60–90 diastolic dipole with a 30-mV baseline depression followed by Q, R, S-T, as seen in the presence of subepicardial injury (Figs. I–88 and I–95).

We can generalize on these S-T baseline phenomena: whenever the damaged (less positively charged) cells are adjacent to the electrode or are sandwiched between normal cells and the electrode, an apparent S-T elevation will be seen. Whenever normal cells are sandwiched between the severely injured cells and the electrode, there will be an illusory S-T depression. Thus, an opposite-wall transmural injury will produce the same S-T depression as an adjacent wall subendocardial injury (Fig. I–96).

In both situations, the dipole is generated by normal cells interspaced between damaged cells and the electrode. With opposite-wall subendocardial injury and adjacent-wall subepicardial injury, the dipole is generated by the damaged cells lying between the electrode and normal cells, and the illusion of S-T elevation is seen (Fig. I–86).

Because the S-T segment in these situations represents that period when there is *no dipole,* the S-T segment remains at true zero throughout and is therefore **horizontal.** This characteristic is of great importance in recognizing acutely injured cells (see later discussion).

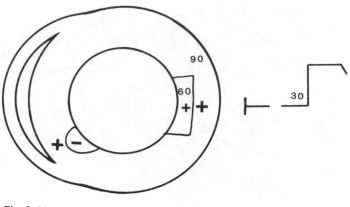

Fig. I–91

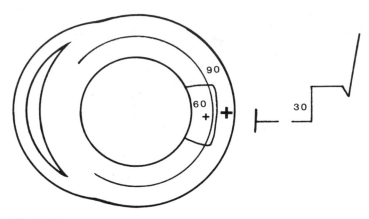

Fig. I–92

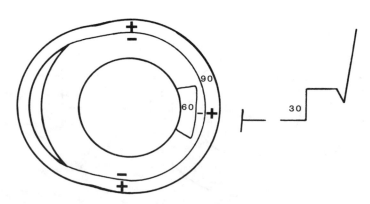

Fig. I–93

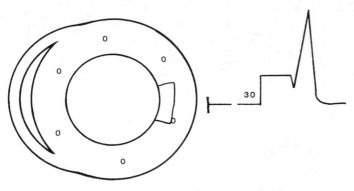

Fig. I–94

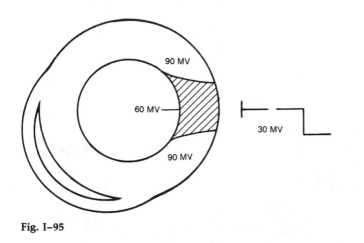

Fig. I–95

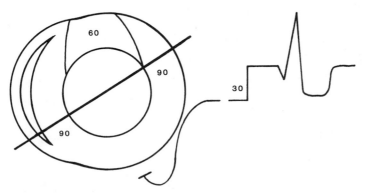

Fig. I–96

MYOCARDIAL INFARCTION

With necrosis, loss of dipoles occurs during depolarization and repolarization. Figure I–97 represents a lateral myocardial loss. During the first .01 and .02 sec, septal depolarization occurs normally and generates a negative deflection in the left-sided lead shown. At .04 seconds, the loss of positively charged dipoles facing left causes the lateral wall to have fewer dipoles than the opposite wall, despite the fact that the opposite wall normally generates fewer dipoles, as has been discussed. Let us again suggest that the opposite wall at .04 sec produces 0.5 million dipoles and the adjacent wall, because of necrotic loss, generates only .2 million. The negative poles of the opposite wall at .04 sec outnumber the positive poles facing the electrode on the adjacent wall; thus, the deflection is negative .3 million units. At .05 to .08 sec, the deficit in positive poles facing the electrode produces the V-shaped QS seen in Figure I–98. The nadir of the V occurs when the inequality is greatest, as shown in Figure I–97.

When loss of the wall involves only the inner layers (Fig. I–98), the deficit is evident during those time intervals when the infarcted strata would have been involved in depolarization. Once the movement of dipoles has advanced to the surviving superficial layers at .05 sec or later, dipole generation reappears and a smaller than normal R wave follows the Q wave.

Three comments may be made about this R wave: (1) it follows a pathologic (.04-sec or greater) Q wave; (2) it is small because of loss of dipole-producing tissue; and (3) it may be delayed by a circuitous route of depolarization wave around or through the infarcted myocardium.

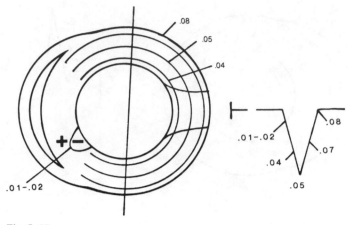

Fig. I–97

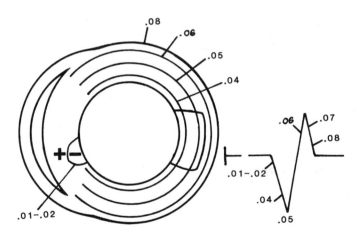

Fig. I–98

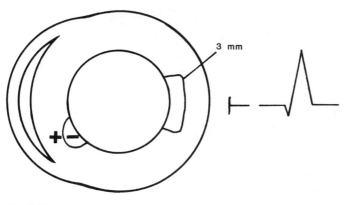

Fig. I–99

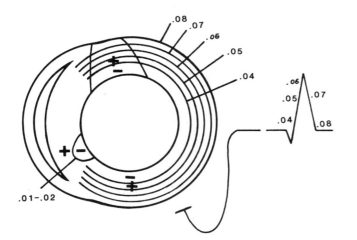

Fig. I–100

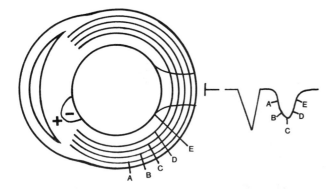

REPOLARIZATION

Fig. I–101

A special situation arises when the necrotic area involves only that subendocardial layer that is normally self-cancelled (Figs. I–26 and I–99). Because this layer makes no contribution to the generation of the normal QRS, its absence has no effect on the QRS. Thus, infarction 3 mm or so deep into the subendocardial myocardium does not produce Q-wave evidence of tissue loss. If, however, the lesion is in the basal subendocardium where there are no Purkinje filaments and hence no self-cancellation, pathologic Q waves can be expected.

Infarction of the wall opposite to an electrode predictably magnifies the R wave (Fig. I–100), because positively oriented dipoles of the healthy adjacent wall are less counterbalanced than normal by the negatively oriented dipoles of the opposite wall.

T WAVES IN INFARCTION

Loss of myocardium also disturbs the balance of dipoles in repolarization (Fig. I–101). As was illustrated in Figure I–73, loss of adjacent wall causes the negative poles of the opposite wall to outnumber the positive charges of the repolarizing damaged adjacent wall.

T waves in subendocardial infarction may be symmetrically inverted or may be diphasic, with the initial portion normally upright and the later portion inverted. Two possibilities could account for a *symmetrically* inverted T. On the one hand, if the more superficial myocardium lying over the subendocardial infarction is damaged and generates *prolonged* action potentials, the "race" between adjacent and opposite walls would go to the opposite wall at each stratum from epicardium to endocardium: the superficial, damaged but surviving, layer would "lose" because of pathologically prolonged (and thus delayed) repolarization, while the infarcted layer would "lose" because of dipole loss. On the other hand, if action potentials of ischemic living cells interspersed among necrotic *subendocardial* cells are pathologically *short*, the adjacent wall would, in repolarization, generate a dipole directed negatively toward the electrode (Fig. I–102). Thus, two diametrically opposed mechanisms can be proposed to explain the symmetrically inverted T wave of subendocardial damage. Evidence that the action potentials of damaged cells are prolonged is derived from the fact that myocardial disease is most frequently associated with extension of the Q-T interval even when QRS duration is not prolonged. More direct evidence of shortening and lengthening of the action potential of injured cells comes from intracellular electrophysiologic studies. The diphasic T waves sometimes seen in subendocardial infarction can best be accounted for by attributing the terminal inversion to prolongation of the action potential of subendocardial cells or to the loss of those cells.

S-T SEGMENT IN INFARCTION

An acute infarction encloses a heterogeneous population of dead cells, severely injured cells with low resting potentials, and less severely injured cells with normal resting potentials but pathologically lengthened or shortened action potentials. The severely damaged cells generate a diastolic dipole, as was discussed earlier. Thus, a transmural infarction with severely injured but surviving cells in its matrix will depress the base line and create the illusion of S-T elevation that has been described (Figs. I–102, I–103). If,

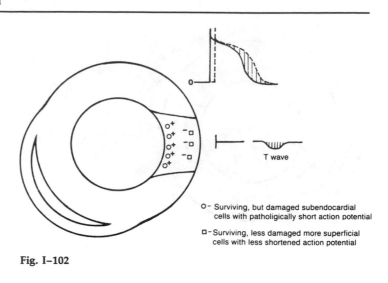

T wave

O – Surviving, but damaged subendocardial cells with pathologically short action potential

□ – Surviving, less damaged more superficial cells with less shortened action potential

Fig. I–102

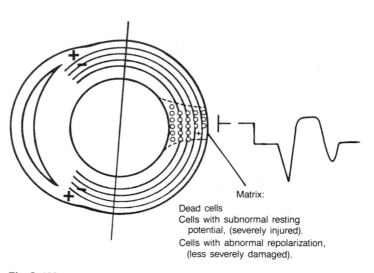

Matrix:
Dead cells
Cells with subnormal resting potential, (severely injured).
Cells with abnormal repolarization, (less severely damaged).

Fig. I–103

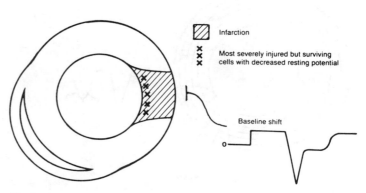

Infarction

Most severely injured but surviving cells with decreased resting potential

Baseline shift

Fig. I–104

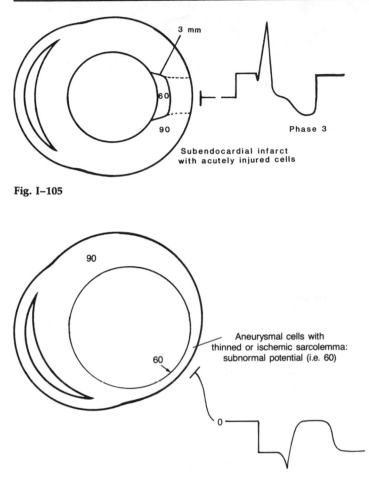

Fig. I–105

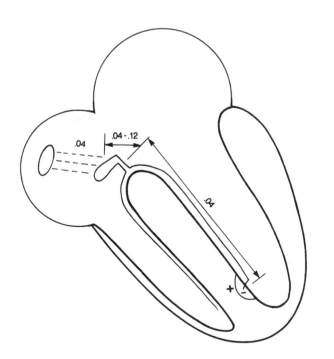

Fig. I–106

by chance, the majority of such cells is deep in the wall, illusory S-T depression will occur (Fig. I–104). S-T depression without pathologic Q wave is expected to be seen in leads overlying subendocardial infarction (Fig. I–105).

Because severely injured cells are not likely to remain in such a precarious state, these cells predictably die or recover. The S-T deviation of acute infarction, therefore, is valuable in estimating the age of the process. Q waves and inverted T waves, on the other hand do not, without serial records, indicate the age of the process, because loss of cells 10 minutes or 10 years old may generate the same Q and T abnormalities.

On occasion, the S-T segment may remain elevated or depressed with the horizontal configuration of acute injury. Most commonly, this phenomenon occurs in the presence of aneurysmal deformity of an infarction; in that situation, the layer of residual myocardial cells is stretched and sarcolemma is thinned, creating a chronic subnormality of resting potential (Fig. I–106) and the illusion of S-T elevation.

A-V CONDUCTION DISORDERS

Conduction from the sinus node to the atrioventricular node normally requires approximately 40 msec (Fig. I–107).

Some evidence suggests that poorly demarcated pathways connect the sinus and A-V nodes and afford more rapid conduction than the contractile atrial myocardium. Transmission of an impulse from the lower A-V node to the interventricular septum also normally takes approximately 40 msec. A significant delay zone occurs at the A-V node, where slow conduction normally requires .04 to .12 sec for passage through the

Fig. I–107

node. The "built-in" delay appears to serve as a means of avoiding contraction of the ventricles before diastolic filling is accomplished. The A-V node may provide desirably slow conduction because of the concentration of Ca^{++} dependent, slow-current cells. Cells that depolarize slowly (Fig. I–108), conduct slowly. The rate of phase-0 depolarization is proportional to the rate of linear conduction.

The A-V nodal region is heavily innervated with sympathetic and parasympathetic nerves that modify depolarization and conduction, as seen in Figure I–109. With increasing vagal tone, conduction and phase 0 are progressively slowed and finally fail to reach transmission threshold. This represents a single-cell phenomenon comparable to Wenckebach block, where the P-R interval increases progressively until finally an atrial impulse is not conducted into the ventricles. If sympathetic stimulation occurs, the reverse occurs, with more and more rapid phase-0 depolarization and more rapid conduction.

The P-R interval represents the time elapsed from the initial depolarization of the peri-sinus atrial myocardium until the first "beachhead" is established on the interventricular septum. Normally, this is .12 to .20 sec. Prolongation of the P-R interval without nonconducted beats (first-degree A-V block) may reflect a delay at any point from sinus node to the septum. If nonconducted beats (second-degree A-V block) occur in the presence of Wenckebach phenomenon, the dysfunction may lie in the heavily innervated A-V node where fluctuation of vagal and sympathetic tone may contribute to the rapid variation of conduction. The response of Wenckebach block to vagolytic or sympathicomimetic drugs appears to substantiate this possibility. Success with these agents usually

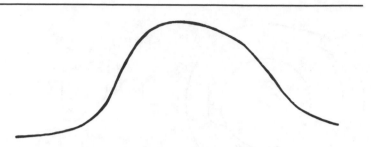

Fig. I–108

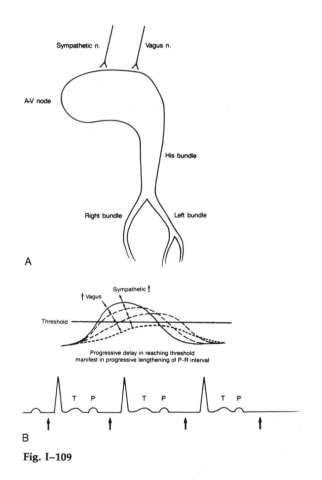

Fig. I–109

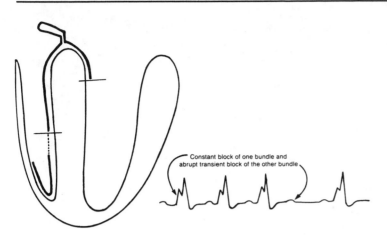

Constant block of one bundle and
abrupt transient block of the other bundle

Fig. I–110

makes it unnecessary to install an extrinsic pacemaker in these patients. Because the A-V node most frequently derives its blood supply from the same vessel that supplies the diaphragmatic posterior myocardium (the right coronary artery), Wenckebach A-V block, when associated with infarction, is most often seen with diaphragmatic-posterior lesions.

Intermittent interruption of A-V conduction may be the result of dysfunction of the right and left bundle branches. This form of A-V block is particularly treacherous because it may come on without warning and may produce complete A-V block and ventricular standstill. It is seen in the presence of bundle branch block that is abruptly complicated by interruption of conduction over the remaining bundle branch system. Thus, a patient with chronic left or right bundle branch block may abruptly develop block in the opposite bundle, leading to complete A-V dissociation (Fig. I–110).

This phenomenon, commonly called Mobitz II block, does not respond to vagolytic agents because the vagus nerve does not innervate the ventricles below the uppermost portion of the interventricular septum. Because of the unpredictable nature of this phenomenon, insertion of an extrinsic pacemaker may be an essential therapeutic measure to protect the patient from abrupt development of persistent complete A-V block with hazardous ventricular bradycardia or standstill.

HEMIBLOCK

The electrocardiographic manifestations of left and right bundle branch block have been discussed. If the interruption of conduction occurs below the bifurcation of the left bundle, left anterior or left posterior hemiblock ensues (Fig. I–111).

As seen in Fig. I–111, conduction over the left posterior hemibranch and the right bundle branch in the presence of left anterior hemiblock leads to depolarization of the posteroseptal and posterior wall in a normal fashion and depolarization of the right side of the septum in normal fashion. The wave of depolarization advances circumferentially through the anteroseptal region, anterior wall, and lateral wall. As this depolarizing dipole moves as shown in Fig. I–111, the positive leading edge of the dipole passes in front of the vantage point of the leads V_1 through V_6 sequentially, while the negative trailing edge of the posterior dipoles faces those leads throughout posterior-wall depolarization. Thus, in V_1 the initial deflection may be a small R wave or a negative wave, depending on the relative dipole strength facing V_1 in the septum and facing away from V_1 in the posterior wall. In successive leads V_2 through V_4 or V_5, the initial deflection should be a small R wave followed by a large negative S wave, which is the product of the trailing edge of anterior- and posterior-wall dipoles. Only in leads placed laterally (V_6, V_7, or V_8) is a predominant upright deflection generated by the positive edges of dipoles advancing through the anterolateral wall and posterior wall. As shown in Fig. I–111, the result is a slow development of R waves as leads are positioned more and more leftward. As will be seen in the later discussion of V leads, this phenomenon has been described as poor progression of R waves or clockwise rotation. As seen in Fig. I–111, the dipole front advances from the terminal filaments of the posterior hemibranch and the right bundle branches, with

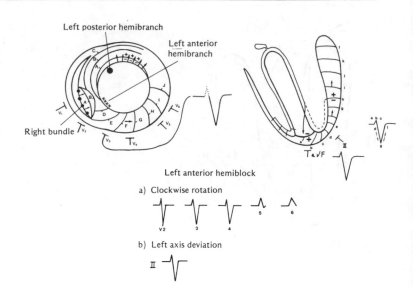

Fig. I–111

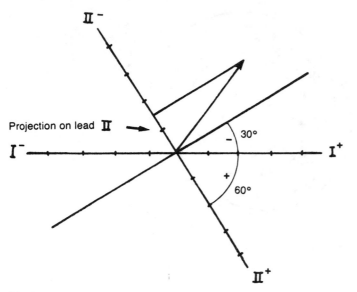

Fig. I–112

its positive aspect facing inferiorly; in the absence of the left anterior hemibranch filaments, conduction into the anterior and lateral wall occurs without benefit of specialized conducting tissue and moves from cell-to-cell in a neighbor-to-neighbor fashion. As a result, the dipole front moves not in a sunburst as is seen in normal persons, but in an apex-to-base sequence. Thus, leads positioned below the heart, especially leads II and aVF, register initial, positive deflections generated by the positive aspect of the early dipoles, followed by large negative deflections generated by the trailing negative aspect of the free-wall dipoles.

The term left axis deviation is usually applied when the QRS complex in lead II is more downward than upward, indicating a negative net vector, as seen in lead II. If, for example, the initial R wave in lead II is 1 mm in height and the S wave in lead II is −3 mm in depth, the net vector is −2. In a stylized human model, the axis of lead II extending from the left leg to the right arm lies 60° below horizontal (Fig. I–112). The projection of a vector on the negative limb of lead II must, as seen in Figure I–112, indicate that the vector lies at an angle greater than −30° above horizontal (above lead I). Left anterior hemiblock can be recognized, therefore, in the presence of (a) clockwise rotation as shown in Figure I–111, and (b) left axis deviation as indicated in Figure I–111 and Figure I–112 and (c) an initial small R wave in lead aVF. The QRS duration may remain within normal limits or may be prolonged slightly in the presence of hemiblock. Because the apical portion of the ventricles depolarizes first in the presence of left anterior hemiblock, repolarization likewise begins in the apical region. As a result, repolarization dipoles generate upright T waves in the inferior leads aVF and II. Also because repolarization of the septum precedes that of the lateral wall (as seen in Fig. I–113), the T waves in left anterior hemiblock are generally upright in right precordial leads and generally flat or inverted in left lateral leads.

Left posterior hemiblock is a rare phenomenon, unlike the commonplace anterior hemiblock. Its electrocardiographic presentation can be visualized as in Figure I–114. As can be seen, the delayed depolarization of the posterior septum and posterior wall leads to a delayed dipole population moving to the right and posteriorly generating terminal negative (S) waves in lead I and prominent late R waves in lead III.

Because right axis deviation can be defined as a more negative than positive QRS deflection in lead I, left posterior hemiblock is one of many causes for right axis deviation. Its presentation is nonspecific, because tall, thin individuals, patients with right ventricular enlargement, and those with loss of the left lateral wall by infarction may equally well present with marked right axis deviation.

The combination of left anterior hemiblock and right bundle branch block is a common occurrence in which the diagnostic features of right bundle branch block are retained (RsR' in V_1, S wave in I and V_6) and left axis deviation is superimposed as a result of the left anterior hemiblock.

COMPLETE HEART BLOCK

As indicated by loss of temporal association of QRS complexes and P waves, atrial rhythm may originate in the sinus node or in an ectopic atrial focus; whereas ventricular rhythm may originate in the junction, bundle

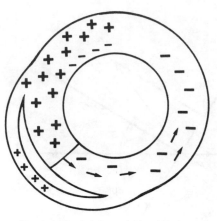

Repolarization in left anterior hemi block

Fig. I–113

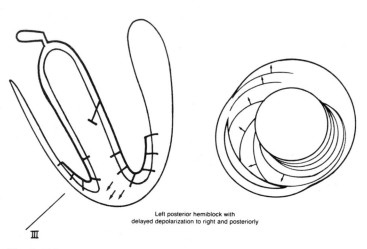
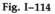

Left posterior hemiblock with
delayed depolarization to right and posteriorly

III

Fig. I–114

of His, bundle branches, or the ventricular myocardium. If the ventricular pacemaker lies in the junction, the QRS, ST-T configuration will appear normal. The ventricular rate may be moderately depressed. Indeed, especially in young individuals with congenital complete A-V block, the ventricular rate may range from 60 to 80 with normal QRS, ST-T configuration. In general, the more distally the pacemaker is located in the ventricle, the less rapid the rate. Ventricular rhythms generated beneath the branching of the common bundle are manifested by wide QRS complexes resembling those seen in bundle branch block. Generally, the sinus rate exceeds ventricular rate. One of the most difficult distinctions may be between complete A-V block and a high degree of second-degree A-V block. Because in the latter instance the ventricular rate may be slow, it is essential to demonstrate the lack of association between atrial and ventricular rhythm. This is done best usually by recognizing the regular cadence of the R-R intervals in the presence of a variable P-R interval in complete A-V block. In the presence of high-degree second-degree A-V block, ventricular rhythm by necessity will be irregular.

A word might be added to clarify "interference dissociations." Classically, this term was used to indicate the situation in which the ventricular rhythm is independent of atrial rhythm and the ventricular rate intermittently exceeds the atrial rate. This phenomenon represents two pacemakers firing at almost the same rate. P waves variably precede, follow, or are lost in the QRS. Although the ventricular pacemaker may lie at any position in the ventricular myocardium, most often it is found in the A-V node, and ventricular complexes are normal. Studies have demonstrated the existence of retrograde block at the A-V node preventing capture of atria by the junctional pacemaker. Antegrade block of the sinus beats occurs as the atrial depolarization advances into the refractory period of the A-V node. The hallmarks of this phenomenon are (1) the ventricular rate slightly exceeds the atrial rate during a portion of each episode, and the P waves and QRS are in *close proximity*, thus distinguishing this from A-V block, in which ventricular rate is seldom greater than the atrial, and the P waves do not persistently "hover" about the QRS; (2) the episodes are self-limited and almost always are free of undesirable hemodynamic consequences; (3) no therapy is required; and (4) there is often no evidence of heart disease.

ATRIAL ARRHYTHMIAS

As seen in Figure I–115a, a normal sinus beat recorded from a left-sided position (I, aVL, V$_5$ through V$_6$) should register a positive deflection during atrial depolarization. In many normal individuals, the P wave presents a shallow dimple at its midpoint as the depolarization wave moves across the interatrial septum.

If, as illustrated in Figure I–115b, an ectopic atrial beat is generated in the left border of the left atrium and advances toward the right atrium, the P wave recorded by the left-sided lead will be an upside-down image of the normal P wave, generated by the negative aspect of the retreating dipole. Repetitive automatic firing of this pacemaker would generate a succession of cookie-cutter look-alike inverted P waves, with a flat horizontal diastolic period between beats (Fig. I–115c). This rhythm would be classified as atrial tachycardia.

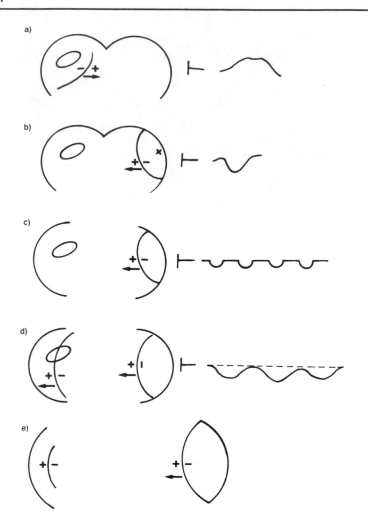

Fig. I–115

If, however, the rate of repetitive firing was such that the preceding beat had not completed its migration before the successive beat was initiated, the lead would record a constantly fluctuating negativity with no quiet diastolic period between beats (Fig. I–115d). This rhythm would resemble precisely what is seen in atrial flutter.

The loss of a rest period between successive beats may be generated by an increased rate of pacemaker firing or it may be induced by slow conduction across the atria without further acceleration of the automatic pacemaker discharge. Likewise, the flutter-like picture with no rest period between atrial beats could be generated in the presence of atrial enlargement, as seen in Figure I–115e. Thus, a patient might present an electrocardiographic record that would be classified as atrial tachycardia at a rate of 180 beats per minute. Another patient, also with an atrial rate of 180 with an impairment of intraatrial conduction, would present a flutter-like configuration, as would a patient with atrial enlargement who had a rate of 180 beats per minute; whereas a patient with normal atrial conduction and normal atrial size would generate a flutter-like configuration only if the atrial rate increased significantly.

Although a rapid atrial rhythm with constantly undulating wave form may be the result of a rapid ectopic focus, classic observations show that this may not necessarily be so. A stimulus applied at any point on a ring preparation of the auricle of the large ray, a cold-blooded animal, starts a wave in each direction; the clockwise and counterclockwise waves meet at the opposite side of the ring and die out. When, however, several stimuli are applied in rapid succession, on some occasions, the wave moves in one direction while tissue in the opposite direction remains refractory (Fig. I–116). The conducted wave advances around the ring sufficiently slowly for the refractory state to wear off. The wave thus continues in a circular fashion for many revolutions. Recordings made with a remote electrode produced flutter-type undulations (Fig. I–116). An essential feature of this laboratory study was the rapidity of the rate of stimulation. Under these conditions, circular conduction appears when, by chance, in the presence of a rapid series of depolarizations, there is inequality of the duration of the refractory period.

Other means of inducing one-way conduction have been achieved in warm-blooded animals. When the dog auricle is stimulated at the insertion of the vena cava, the wave fronts advance clockwise and counterclockwise around the cava and are extinguished upon collision on the opposite side. When conduction through the intercaval myocardium is blocked permanently by crushing of this tissue, or temporarily by application of cocaine, stimulation of the nearby atrial myocardium produces one-way advance of the depolarization wave around the cavae. When cocaine block subsides in 1 to 2 minutes, bidirectional conduction reappears and the circular rhythm subsides. In the warm-blooded animal, as in the ray, flutter-like rhythms can be produced by very rapid atrial stimulation. The phenomenon appears to be caused by a lack of homogeneity of the refractory period and is facilitated by a rapid rate of stimulation.

The possibility that focal stimulation of the atria may elicit a train of afterpotentials sufficiently large to reach threshold and generate a triggered rhythm must be considered. If the resulting triggered rhythm were sufficiently rapid to cause each succeeding depolarization to begin its advance before the

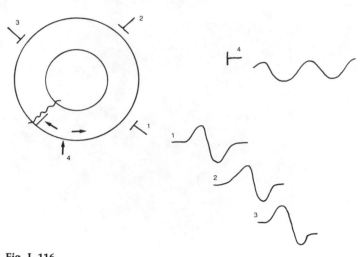

Fig. I–116

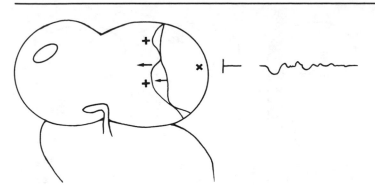

Fig. I–117

preceding wave front had run its course, a remote electrode would record a flutter-like phenomenon as illustrated in Figure I–115d and e. Generally, an atrial tachycardia with isoelectric baseline between atrial waves will be classified atrial tachycardia. The rate will most often be less than 220 beats per minute. When the atrial rhythm is regular, without an isoelectric period between beats, and with a rate between 250 and 350 beats per minute, the record is usually designated as flutter. Clearly, the clinical distinction between atrial tachycardia and atrial flutter can be an arbitrary one.

Often there is a progressive acceleration of the rate during the "warm-up" period of an ectopic atrial tachycardia. Possibly, this can be attributed to failure of the sarcolemmal pump to keep up with the burden of sodium and potassium transport, with a resultant shift of the transmembrane potential toward threshold. Stabilization of the rate after "warm-up" may reflect an equilibrium between Na-K transport requirements and sarcolemmal function.

If a focus in the atrium is firing so rapidly that its irregular trailing edge is overtaken by the succeeding beat in an irregular fashion, the net wave front would be a constantly changing negative deflection as illustrated in Figure I–117.

Thus, each of the recognized atrial arrhythmias theoretically may be generated by an ectopic focus. Fibrillation appears when the rate of ectopic discharge is so rapid that an irregular, constantly changing block of succeeding beats occurs.

Although atrial arrhythmias may be initiated from any portion of the atria, the A-V node is especially important in the genesis of atrial arrhythmia because of the functional characteristics of its cells. One family of junctional cells is characterized by slow conduction and a short refractory period; whereas another type of cell conducts rapidly, with a long "tail" of refractoriness. These dual pathways may be likened to two railroad trains on parallel tracks, one a long fast train and one a slow short train. These "tracks" are interconnected by lateral pathways at intervals. As seen in Figure I–118, an atrial premature beat approaching the junction may fall on the rapid conducting pathway in its refractory state when the slowly conducting path is no longer refractory.

An impulse may then progress down the slow path and reach a transverse interconnection which is no longer refractory. The depolarization could enter the fast path and move retrograde into the upper junction and into the atria, producing a reentry atrial beat. The depolarizing wave front, as seen in Figure I–119, may then reenter the now-receptive slow path and complete the circuit within the junction.

Atrial and ventricular beats are produced as the wave front revolves between the His bundle and the atrial myocardial cells. The circuit may be enclosed within the A-V node or may include a portion of the atrial myocardium (Fig. I–120). To be sustained, the reentry rhythm requires a nonrefractory population of cells into which the dipole can advance. It is generally believed that most episodes of supraventricular tachycardia are a result of this reentry process.

If the antegrade conduction advances along the slow tract and returns retrograde by way of the fast tract, atrial depolarization occurs during ventricular depolarization and the P wave is lost within the QRS complex. This is the most common form of reentry supraventricular tachycardia. A paroxysm of reen-

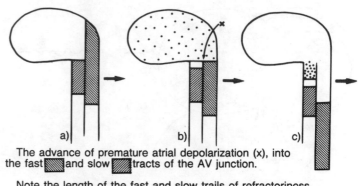

The advance of premature atrial depolarization (x), into the fast ▨ and slow ▨ tracts of the AV junction.

Note the length of the fast and slow trails of refractoriness.

Fig. I–118

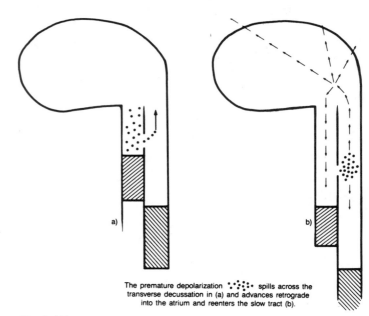

The premature depolarization ⁛ spills across the transverse decussation in (a) and advances retrograde into the atrium and reenters the slow tract (b).

Fig. I–119

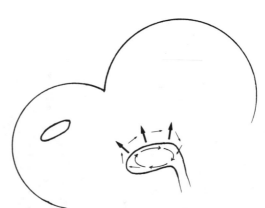

Fig. I–120

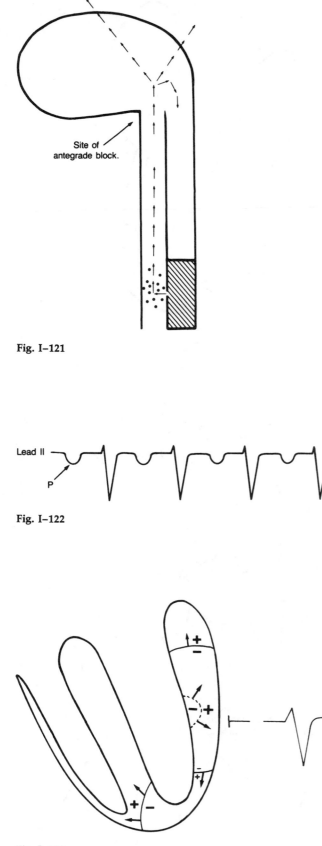

Fig. I–121

Lead II

P

Fig. I–122

Fig. I–123

try tachycardia is most readily precipitated by an atrial premature contraction that reaches the A-V node at a time when the slow and fast "trains" are leaving the nodal "station" as shown in Figure I–118 and I–119. This requires *precise* timing. Thus, most atrial premature contractions arrive when both tracts, the slow and the fast, are either refractory or are both prepared to conduct; it is much more likely that an atrial premature beat will be blocked or will be conducted normally through the junction than that it will arrive at the unique time when the unequal refractoriness of the slow and fast tracts will initiate the reentry phenomenon.

Less commonly, antegrade conduction through the A-V node may proceed by way of the fast tract, with retrograde conduction over the slow pathway. This phenomenon is less easily visualized. Perhaps antegrade block at the upper portion of the slow tract with transverse decussion lying low in the His bundle may set up the situation as seen in Figure I–121.

Depolarization would proceed retrograde over the slow tract to the atria. Whatever the mechanism, the electrocardiographic result is the occurrence of a retrograde P wave long after the QRS (Fig. I–122). For unknown reasons, this phenomenon is persistent and has been called "incessant tachycardia," lasting for prolonged periods, interrupted by short periods of normal rhythm. This phenomenon is especially frequent in children and is often refractory to therapy.

VENTRICULAR ARRHYTHMIAS

If a Purkinje cell located as shown in Figure I–123 reaches threshold by spontaneous depolarization, the dipole can be expected to advance into the myocardium. The initial process will expand into the neighboring myocardium and generate an initial R wave in a lead recorded as shown. Subsequently, the wave front will advance in domino fashion through the myocardium and may also advance in a retrograde direction over the bundle branch, as shown in Figure I–124. As a result, the terminal portion of the QRS in an overlying lead will be a negative (S) deflection. The duration of the QRS will be determined by the time required to reach and depolarize the most distant myocardium. If the process advances through nonspecialized myocardium, the QRS will be significantly prolonged; whereas conduction of the process over the rapidly conducting Purkinje system will result in a less drastically prolonged QRS. Clearly, cardiac enlargement would prolong the conduction process under either circumstance. The "birthplace" of a premature ventricular contraction (PVC) can therefore be recognized by finding that lead which shows a small initial R followed by a large S wave. Because this area depolarizes first, it will repolarize first, generating an upright T wave in the overlying lead.

Repetitive discharge of a subendocardial ventricular focus may produce couplets, triplets, or when more than three in a row, ventricular tachycardia. Sharply defined QRS complexes are formed when depolarization expands over normally conducting myocardial or Purkinje cells (Fig. I–125). When, however, the rate of sodium entry (phase 0), is slowed by reduction of electrical gradient by ischemia or electrolyte disorder or by drugs, the QRS generated by the ectopic beat is more prolonged and less sharply inscribed (Fig. I–126).

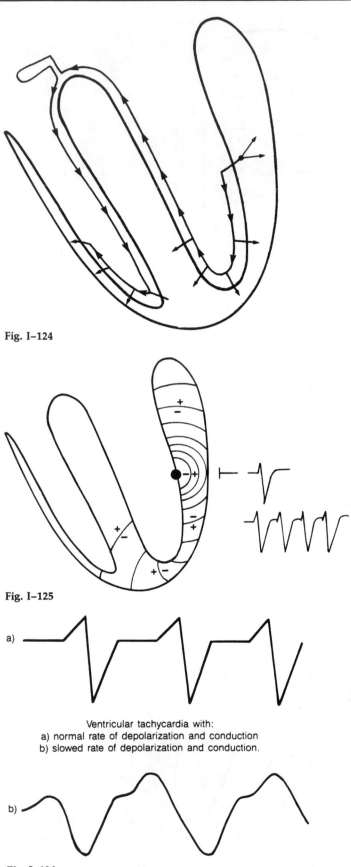

Fig. I–124

Fig. I–125

a)

Ventricular tachycardia with:
a) normal rate of depolarization and conduction
b) slowed rate of depolarization and conduction.

b)

Fig. I–126

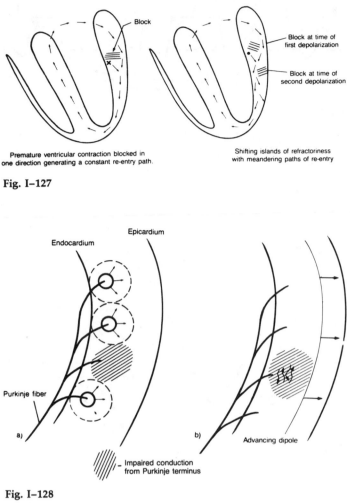

Premature ventricular contraction blocked in one direction generating a constant re-entry path.

Shifting islands of refractoriness with meandering paths of re-entry

Fig. I–127

Fig. I–128

Impaired conduction from Purkinje terminus

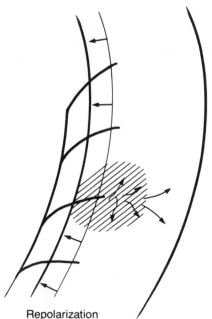

Repolarization

Fig. I–129

When conduction from the initiating focus is severely and irregularly impaired, a beat-to-beat variation in the depolarizing wave front results in varying QRS configurations. Should the impairment of conduction in one direction block the advance of depolarization, the stage is set for circuitous reentry phenomenon with a chaotic, meandering path and disorganized activation of the myocardium. Thus, the occurrence of fibrillation, as well as all varieties of ventricular tachyarrhythmias, may be unifocal in onset (Fig. I–127).

Because all these arrhythmias may be unifocal does not mean they *must* be so. Indeed, it is likely that many ventricular premature contractions, especially those with a fixed time relation to the preceding normal beat (fixed coupling) are the result of a reentry of the depolarizing wave front. As shown in Figure I–128, interruption of the conduction from Purkinje terminals into a small area of the syncytium of subendocardial myocardial cells may produce a labyrinthine depolarizing path (Fig. I–129). When the time of conduction of this micro-reentry process exceeds the refractory period of the surrounding normally conducting tissue, the depolarization wave may exit from the labyrinth and invade the neighboring myocardium, with ensuing QRS configuration as produced from a unifocal depolarization. Thus, the electrocardiographic appearance of the QRS and S-T,T does not distinguish a premature, unifocal, depolarization from a depolarization initiated by a small area of re-entry (micro-reentry).

When ventricular premature contractions occur at a regular interval unrelated to the time of occurrence of normal beats, an independent focus shielded from the remainder of the myocardium exists, resembling an independent kingdom surrounded by a moat. Control of traffic across the bridge over the moat determines the resulting rhythm. If entering traffic is blocked (entrance block) but the exit is unimpaired, premature contractions will occur in response to each depolarization of "the castle." If exit traffic progressively slows to the point of total block, the occurrence of the premature contraction is progressively delayed and finally fails to occur. This represents Wenckebach second-degree exit block and can be recognized as seen in Figure I–130. If entry traffic is only intermittently blocked, the independent kingdom, properly called a parasystolic focus, intermittently ceases to originate ectopic beats because invasion of the "kingdom" leads to depolarization of the focus before it can spontaneously reach threshold.

If the site of the automatic focus or of the micro-reentry were to migrate during a run of ventricular tachycardia, the QRS configuration would vary; or if there were a fluctuating length of refractory period, the course of depolarization-invasion of the myocardium would vary. Under either circumstance, prolongation of the refractory period would facilitate the variation in depolarization (Fig. I–131). This phenomenon yields a progressively changing QRS configuration during ventricular tachycardia, which has been called torsade de pointes (turning of the points) (Fig. I–132). This is known to occur in the presence of prolongation of Q-T interval, and at times, is precipitated by those Class I anti-arrhythmic drugs which prolong the action potential (and thus the refractory period).

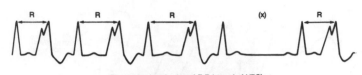

Progressive lengthening of R-R interval of VPC's with non-conducted beat (x) with second degree exit block producing Wenckebach's phenomenon

Fig. I–130

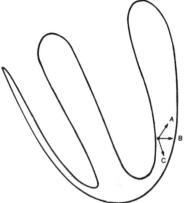

Focus firing every 250 msec:

• First beat advances in sunburst fashion.

• Area A is refractory to second beat, and beat is conducted B+C.

• Third beat is blocked over A+B, and advances in direction of C.

• Fourth beat is blocked over B+C, but conducts in direction A.

Fig. I–131

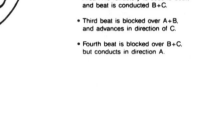

Fig. I–132

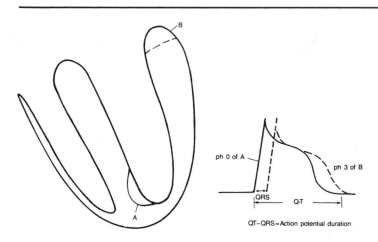

ph 0 of A

ph 3 of B

QRS   Q-T

QT−QRS=Action potential duration

Fig. I–133

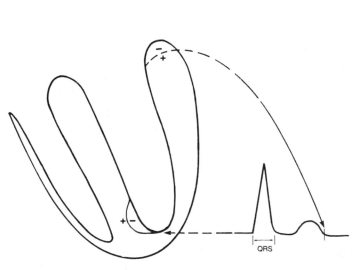

QRS

Fig. I–134

ADDITIONAL RELATIONSHIPS OF THE ACTION POTENTIAL TO THE ELECTROCARDIOGRAM

The initial deflection of the QRS complex is generated by phase 0 of the first ventricular cells to depolarize, and the final portion of the T wave is produced by the terminal portion of phase 3 of the last ventricular cell to repolarize (Fig. I–133).

To determine the duration of a *representative* action potential, it would be necessary to determine the time of phase 0 of the last cell to depolarize or the end of phase 3 of the first cell to repolarize. Because, normally, the last cell (Fig. I–134) to depolarize is also the last to repolarize, and because its phase 0 marks the final component of the QRS complex, the duration of its action potential is measured from the end of the QRS to the end of the T wave. Recognition of this relationship between action potential and EKG has been a significant aid in appreciating the role of single-cell phenomena in the generation of the EKG and illustrates the temporal magnitude of single-cell events.

ELECTROLYTES AND THE ACTION POTENTIAL AND THE ELECTROCARDIOGRAM

Several disorders distort a portion of the action potential and thereby alter the EKG.

Hyperkalemia steepens the slope of phase 3 (potassium exit), which can be remembered simply by recalling the common-sense adage that "if there is more of something, it may perform its action more rapidly." When phase 3 of the ventricular cells becomes steeper, the instantaneous difference in surface charges increases and, as a result, the T wave is taller (Fig. I–135).

Hypokalemia, on the other hand, decreases the slope of phase 3, and thereby flattens the T wave and lengthens the Q-T interval. Indeed, if the deformity of phase 3 is not equally distributed among ventricular cells, inversion of the T wave may occur (Fig. I–136).

Because phase 2 is the time of calcium entry into the cell, the electrocardiographic consequences of hyper- and hypocalcemia are predictable if, once again, one reasons that the more there is of something, the more rapidly it will perform its act. Thus, hypercalcemia shortens phase 2 and hastens its downturn into phase 3 (Fig. I–137). As a result, the hypercalcemic EKG is as seen in Fig. I–138 and resembles the configuration generated by digitalis action. The inter-relation of digitalis effect and sarcolemmal transport of calcium provides a memory-assist for recalling the configuration seen in hypercalcemia. Hypocalcemia, on the other hand, is associated with a long, drawn-out phase 2 and S-T segment. This accordion effect is distinguished from the Q-T prolongation of hypokalemia in that the hypocalcemic Q-T prolongation is a result of S-T lengthening, whereas hypokalemic Q-T prolongation is a result of extension of phase 3 and the T wave. U waves are seen regularly in hypokalemia but are not associated with hypocalcemia (Fig. I–139).

ELECTROCARDIOGRAPHIC "POSITION"

Extremity leads I, II, and III and aVR, aVL and aVF are shown overlying a frontal plane diagram of the heart in Figure I–140. As seen

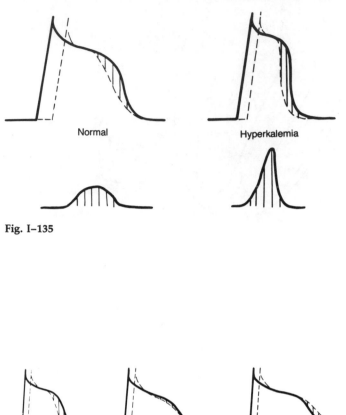

Normal   Hyperkalemia

Fig. I–135

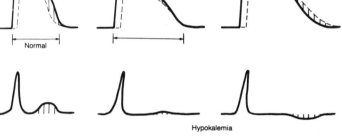

Normal

Hypokalemia

Fig. I–136

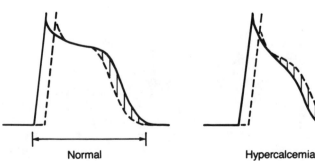

Normal   Hypercalcemia

Fig. I–137

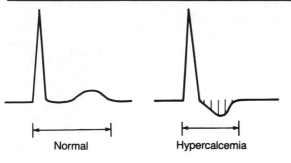

Fig. I–138

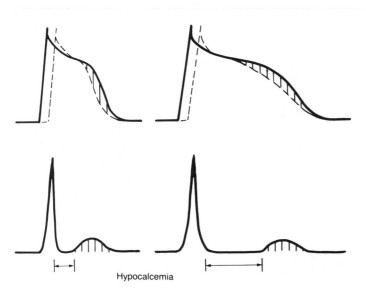

Fig. I–139

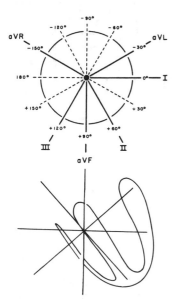
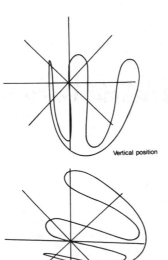

Fig. I–140

in the frontal plane illustration, variation in cardiac position produces predictable QRS, S-T and T configurations in these extremity leads. The cross-sectional, horizontal-plane V leads are seen in Figure I–141. The V leads are best understood by observing the projections of the septal, apical, and left free-wall vectors on the axes of the leads (Fig. I–142A).

As illustrated, septal depolarization, in the first 20 msec of the QRS, produces a right-ward positive vector that generates an initial R wave in V_1. Septal contribution of this R wave grows progressively smaller in V_2 and V_3, while apical (30 msec) depolarization makes an increasing contribution to the initial positive deflection. The free-wall vector, as shown, produces a large negative terminal deflection in V_1, which becomes smaller in V_2 and V_3. Free-wall depolarization then produces an increasingly tall R wave in V_4 through V_6, as illustrated. Thus, the normal V leads show an increasingly tall R wave from V_1 to V_6 (Fig. I–142b). Q waves appear in left-sided leads. As seen in Figure I–143, T waves in the V leads are generated as repolarization is initiated in the apical-septal region, with cell-surface positivity advancing from apex to base. Whether V_1 and V_2 normally register an upright or inverted T wave is determined by the relation of the leads to the septal dipoles. If the septal repolarization lies predominantly cranial to the leads, the positive side of the apical and septal dipole will face V_1 and V_2. If, however, V_1 and V_2 lie near the base of the septum, the negative advancing face of the repolarization dipole will produce a negative T wave in these leads.

QRS configuration in the V leads is subject to considerable normal variation. "Clockwise rotation" with slow progression of R waves from V_1 to V_6 can be the result of simple

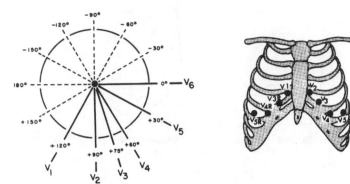

Fig. I–141

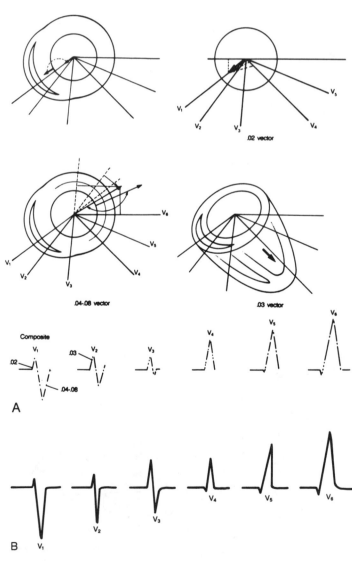

Fig. I–142

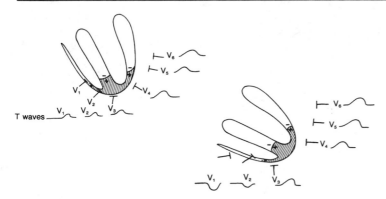

T waves

Fig. I–143

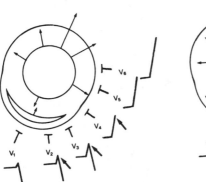

Fig. I–144

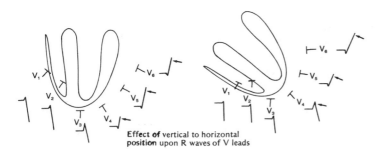

Effect of vertical to horizontal position upon R waves of V leads

Fig. I–145

rotation of the heart about a vertical axis (Fig. I–144) or can be the result of increased horizontal position of the heart (Fig. I–145).

These two mechanisms have been dubbed the "barber-pole" and the "windshield wiper" causes of "poor R wave progression." Another mechanism may be considered: If the initial beachhead of depolarization on the left septal myocardium is located (1) near the base of the ventricles, (2) near the apex, or (3) at the midpoint, the net vector of the septal depolarization may be positively directed toward the base or the apex, as seen in Figure I–146a.

The direction of the free-wall vector is influenced by the degree of extension of the Purkinje net up the free wall, as shown in Figure I–146b. A network that ends near the left ventricular apex would generate a headward vector, with small projections on V_3 through V_6 (poor progression of R waves and left-axis deviation); whereas extension of the Purkinje fibers toward the base would produce free-wall vectors with large projections on V_4 through V_6.

Although variations in Purkinje distribution may account for commonplace variations in "electrical position," anatomic position of the ventricular mass may equally well determine the apparent electrical position (Fig. I–146c).

PERICARDITIS

Sarcolemmal damage produced by inflammation of the epicardial myocardium may increase the entrance to and decrease the extrusion of sodium from these cells. As a result, the increased cation content of the injured cells diminishes their resting potential (Fig. I–147). As seen in Figure I–147, this epicardial process generates a difference in diastolic resting potential. Leads arrayed around the "horseshoe" of the ventricles therefore register a depression of diastolic baseline that is abolished with systolic depolarization, generating the illusion of S-T elevation in all leads except those facing into the cavity of the horseshoe (aVR and, possibly, aVL and V_1). Epicardial damage to the atria may contribute an interesting manifestation of pericarditis, as shown in Figure I–148a, by reducing the diastolic resting potential of epicardial atrial cells.

This (+) aspect of the diastolic dipole of the atria is directed toward all leads except V_1 and aVR; this dipole tends to counterbalance the resting difference in potential generated in the ventricular myocardium. With atrial depolarization, this atrial diastolic dipole is extinguished and the downward displacement of the baseline is accentuated in the interval between atrial and ventricular depolarization. Thus, the illusion of P-R depression is generated.

T-wave inversion in pericarditis is a reflection of the alteration of repolarization of the superficial myocardial cells as a result either of delay in conduction of depolarization into the superficial layers or of pathologic alteration of phase 3 (Fig. I–148b). In either instance, the superficial strata would repolarize after the normal deeper layers, generating a repolarization dipole as shown in Figure I–148b.

NORMAL S-T VARIATIONS

If the resting potential of all ventricular myocardial cells is the same, no illusion of S-T deviation resulting from baseline shift occurs. Or, if there is a random distribution

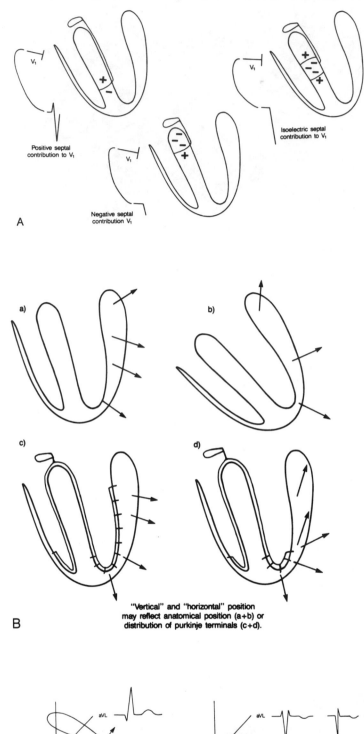

A

Positive septal contribution to V_1

Negative septal contribution V_1

Isoelectric septal contribution to V_1

B

"Vertical" and "horizontal" position may reflect anatomical position (a+b) or distribution of purkinje terminals (c+d).

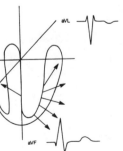

C

Fig. I–146

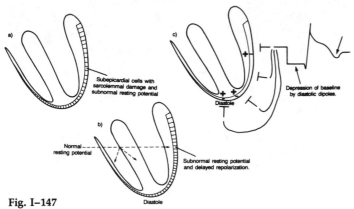

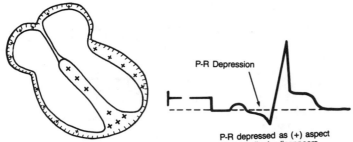

Fig. I–147

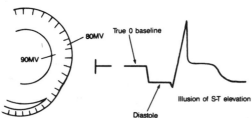

P-R Depression

P-R depressed as (+) aspect
of atrial dipole disappears
with atrial depolarization.

|||| Subepicardial strata of
    decreased resting potential

A

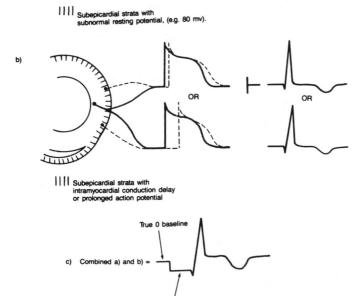

a)

80MV

90MV

True 0 baseline

Illusion of S-T elevation

Diastole

|||| Subepicardial strata with
    subnormal resting potential, (e.g. 80 mv).

b)

OR   OR

|||| Subepicardial strata with
    intramyocardial conduction delay
    or prolonged action potential

True 0 baseline

c) Combined a) and b) =

Diastole

B

Fig. I–148

of cells with varying resting potentials, as indicated in Figure I–149, the mean resting potential in all areas of the ventricular myocardium would be equal and there would be no baseline shift. If, however, the distribution of cells with unequal resting potentials were not random, but instead, the mean resting potential in one area differed from that in another, a diastolic dipole would be generated, a baseline shift would occur, and the illusion of S-T deviation would result.

Apparently, this is a commonplace occurrence in normal individuals. Indeed, the limits of normal S-T deviation reflect this phenomenon and are generally accepted to range from 2 mm elevation to .75 mm depression in precordial leads where proximity produces magnification of wave forms. In some normal individuals, S-T deviations exceed these limits. While inequality of resting potentials may produce these excessive, although normal, variations, alterations in configuration of action potentials may produce equally impressive "normal" S-T and T variation. If phase 2 of the action potential is altered as shown in Figure I–150, the premature recovery of positive surface charge on the cells in area A would generate a dipole during the S-T period that would generate a concave-up S-T elevation in the lead shown and, as indicated in this figure, produce a prominent upright T wave.

These "normal" S-T and T configurations resulting from significant variation in resting potential and/or premature repolarization may be confused with the electrocardiographic signs of pericarditis and epicardial injury. In both situations, S-T elevation is striking; however, the T waves in the normal variant are likely to be impressively tall because of premature recovery of position surface charge in phase 3, whereas the T waves

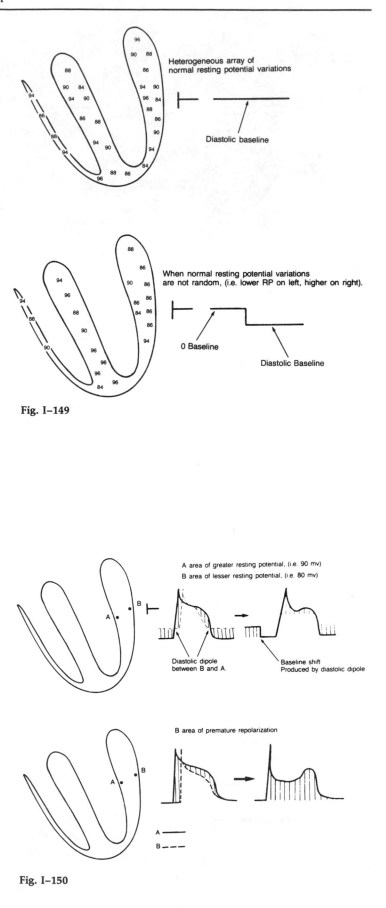

Fig. I–149

Fig. I–150

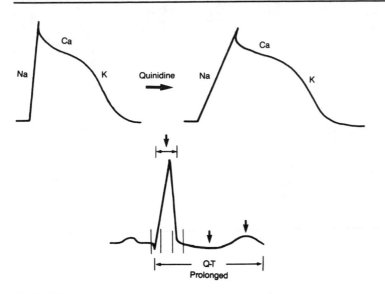

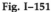

Fig. I–151

in pericarditis are likely to be low or inverted as a result of delay in phase 3 of the action potential of the subepicardial cells.

Most helpful in distinguishing these two processes are the serial changes that occur in the presence of the active pericardial process and the depression of P-R interval seen in pericarditis.

EFFECTS OF DRUGS ON THE ACTION POTENTIAL AND THE ELECTROCARDIOGRAM

Quinidine impedes the movement of sodium, potassium, and calcium across the sarcolemma. With impairment of the rate of Na entry, phase 0 of the action potential is less vertical and conduction is slowed. As a result, the duration of the QRS complex is lengthened by quinidine. Reduction in the rate of Ca entry through sarcolemmal slow-channels is reflected in the prolongation of the plateau of phase 2 and of its derivative, the S-T segment. With slowing of the exit of K, the slope of phase 3 is altered, as shown in Figure I–151, and the T wave, is altered. With prolongation of each component of the action potential and with slowing of conduction, the Q-T interval is a consistent indicator of quinidine effect. Indeed, the most notable changes produced by quinidine are a gentle smoothing of the upstroke and downstroke of the T wave and an accordion-like stretching of the J-T segment (the J point indicating the junction of the QRS complex and the onset of the S-T segment). These effects are seen with therapeutic levels of the drug. Only with large, often toxic, concentrations of quinidine is a prolongation of the QRS complex sufficiently marked to be convincingly measured. A 25% increase in QRS duration after administration of quinidine is often considered to reflect an excess of the drug.

Procainamide, another type I antiarrhythmic drug, resembles quinidine in its effects on sarcolemmal traffic, and therefore produces similar electrocardiographic changes.

Disopyramide similarly decreases the upslope of phase 0 and prolongs the duration of the action potential and generates electrocardiographic changes comparable to those induced by quinidine and procainamide.

Digitalis, unlike the type I drugs that slow transsarcolemmal ionic traffic, acts by impeding the action of the sarcolemmal Na-K ATPase. As a result, the rate of extrusion of Na from the cell is reduced and the active transfer of K into the cell is impeded. The effect of the accumulation of cation (Na) ions and the reduction in rate of reentry of K into the cell is a more rapid net loss of K in late phase 2 and phase 3. The resultant change in configuration of action potential is an increase in downslope of late phase 2 and phase 3. With shortening and down-turning of phases 2 and 3, the S-T,T configuration is altered by digitalis as shown in Figure I–152. Digitalis therefore appears to accelerate some of those events that quinidine delays. Unlike quinidine, however, digitalis has no notable effect on Na entry, phase 0 of the action potential, or intraventricular conduction. Therefore, digitalis does not provoke widening of the QRS complex.

The S-T,T configuration of digitalis effect resembles in some ways that produced by left ventricular hypertrophy. As was noted earlier, left ventricular hypertrophy may be expected to increase the height and width of the QRS. Also to be expected is a change in S-T,T when conduction through the ven-

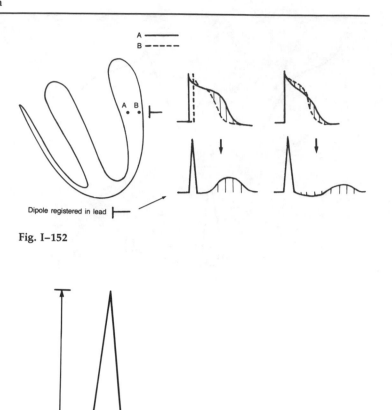

Fig. I–152

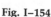

"Full blown" configuration of L.V.H.

Fig. I–153

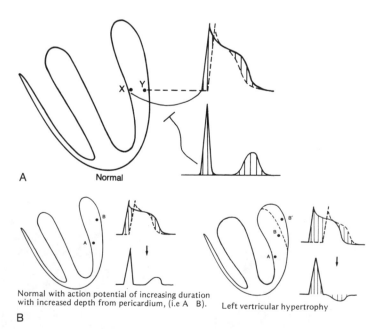

A   Normal

Normal with action potential of increasing duration with increased depth from pericardium, (i.e A B).

B

Left vertricular hypertrophy

Fig. I–154

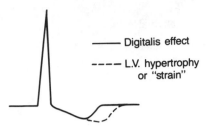

Fig. I-155

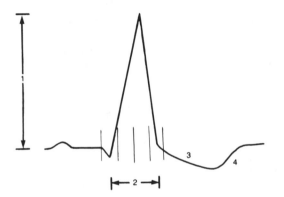

4 Components of classic LV hypertrophy configuration.

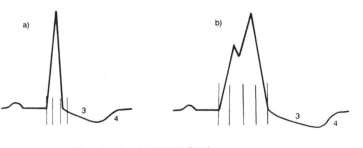

S-T, T configuration of a) LV "strain", and
b) LV conduction delay.

Fig. I-156

tricular myocardium is prolonged by an increase in left ventricular size by dilatation of hypertrophy (Fig. I-153).

If we consider the electrocardiogram to be the composite of the action potentials of all the myocardial cells, we can derive a two-cell model using a subendocardial (long action potential) and a subepicardial (short action potential) cell as was shown in Figures I-66 and I-67.

At each point in time, the difference in potential between the two action potentials is the dipole in existence at that moment (Figs. I-66 and I-67). It is represented by the vertical line connecting simultaneous points of the two action potentials. The action potentials of the normal two-cell heart and the derived electrocardiogram are seen in Figure I-154a. When an intraventricular conduction delay is produced by hypertrophy or dilatation, the effects on the two-cell model are seen as shown in Figure I-154b.

Thus, left ventricular hypertrophy predictably produces an S-T,T deformity with a down-sloping S-T segment rather like that produced by digitalis effect (Fig. I-155). A significant distinction lies in the shortened Q-T interval generated by digitalis effect and the lengthened Q-T duration in the presence of left ventricular hypertrophy. This S-T,T configuration is, in fact, more frequently produced by left ventricular hypertrophy than is the full-blown picture of tall, wide QRS followed by down-sloping S-T segment and "invisible" T wave (Fig. I-156). It has become customary to consider this S-T,T configuration, when associated with a normal QRS complex, to be compatible with left ventricular strain.

Because this configuration results from conduction delay in hypertrophy, it is not surprising to find the same S-T,T form in the presence of other conduction delays, most notably in left bundle branch block.

EFFECTS OF THE NERVOUS SYSTEM ON THE ACTION POTENTIAL AND THE ELECTROCARDIOGRAM

Catecholamines and sympathetic stimulation accelerate the traffic of Na, K, and Ca across the sarcolemma. Predictably, phase 2 (Na + Ca) and phase 3 (K) of the action potential are modified, with shortening and down-sloping of phase 2 and early completion of phase 3 (Fig. I–157a). The two-cell model illustrates the effects of these changes on the electrocardiogram (Fig. I–157b).

The shortened, down-sloping S-T and flattened T waves, which resemble the effects of digitalis on the S-T,T configuration, may be seen in a variety of commonplace sympathomimetic situations, including fright, exercise, and even assumption of a standing position. Acceleration of sodium entry in phase 0 is not generally perceptible because the upstroke of phase 0 is normally so nearly vertical as to preclude notable increase. When depolarization accelerates during phase 4, diastolic depolarization reaches threshold of Na-dependent pacemaker cells, with the frequent occurrence of premature beats. During tachycardia, this phenomenon is potentiated because more rapid ionic traffic in the presence of a rapid heart rate may over-run the Na-K ATPase "pump," with a resultant reduction in transmembrane resting potential. Thus, tachycardia may beget premature beats or more rapid tachycardia.

When sympathomimetic influence is unevenly distributed over the ventricles, interesting electrocardiographic changes occur. If,

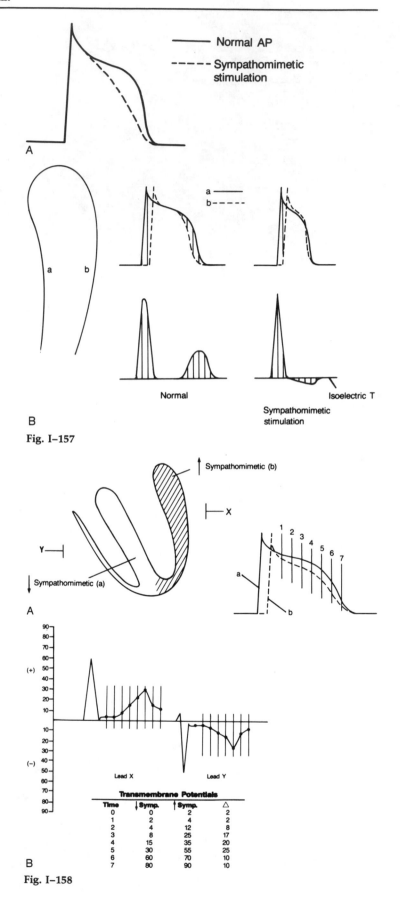

Fig. I–157

Fig. I–158

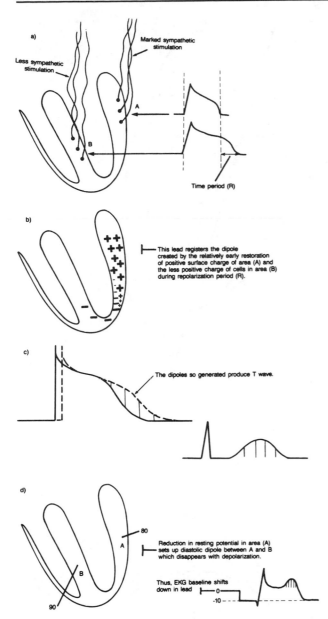

a) Less sympathetic stimulation

Marked sympathetic stimulation

A

B

Time period (R)

b) ++ ++ ++ + + + + + - - -

This lead registers the dipole created by the relatively early restoration of positive surface charge of area (A) and the less positive charge of cells in area (B) during repolarization period (R).

c) The dipoles so generated produce T wave.

d) 80 A B 90

Reduction in resting potential in area (A) sets up diastolic dipole between A and B which disappears with depolarization.

Thus, EKG baseline shifts down in lead. 0 -10

Fig. I–159

for example, one region of the ventricular mass were to be more stimulated than the remainder, that area would be more rapidly repolarized during phases 2 and 3 (Fig. I–158A), and the S-T segment and T waves would be elevated (Fig. I–159).

Such inequality of sympathetic "play" on the myocardium may be responsible for the impressive S-T,T abnormalities produced by a variety of non-cardiac disorders. Notably, afferent impulses from the actively disordered gallbladder may ascend to the vasomotor center and return by sympathetic efferents to the heart. If the sympathetic discharge on the heart is uneven, impressive S-T,T abnormalities may result in the absence of myocardial ischemia (although the possibility of neurogenic coronary spasm must be considered). The S-T,T variations seen in the presence of central nervous system disease appear to be the result of direct, reflex, or internuncial action on the brain stem. Potent, unequal neural influences on the sarcolemma may result in regional variations of resting potential as well as alterations in phases 2, 3, and 4 of the action potential. Significant S-T elevation or depression with striking up- or downslope and magnification, flattening, or inversion of T waves may appear (Fig. I–159).

MEASUREMENT OF TIME INTERVALS AND LIMITS OF NORMAL

The P-R interval represents the time from the "break out" of the depolarization process from the sinus node to the onset of depolarization of the left side of the interventricular septum. This normally requires .12 to .20 sec, of which approximately .04 sec is spent in conduction from the sinus to the A-V node perimeter, and approximately .04 sec from the lower A-V node to the interventricular septum. The remaining .04 to .12 sec are the time of passage through the A-V node.

The mean vector of atrial depolarization is directed from right to left, and it is usually projected clearly on the axis in lead II. The initial septal depolarization vector is directed from left to right and from apex to base, thereby projecting clearly on the axis of lead II. The final ventricular depolarization at the base of the left ventricle is directed headward and it too is projected well on lead II. For these reasons, lead II is usually satisfactory for measurement of P-R and QRS durations (Fig. I–160).

Sometimes, however, the initial atrial depolarization or final basal depolarization is directed at 90° to the axis of lead II and the P-R or QRS duration is falsely foreshortened. It is prudent, therefore, to scan other leads to exclude possible false shortening. If the initial septal depolarization vector lies at 90° to lead II, the P-R interval will be falsely extended in that lead. Once again, it is wise to study other leads to rule out possible error. When precordial leads are used to measure time intervals, often there is a rounding of the initial downslope of Q or of the final downstroke of R or the upstroke of S, because those leads, owing to proximity, record the first and last few cells to depolarize and record those events which may not be registered on the more distant extremity leads. Frequently, therefore, QRS duration may be greater in precordial than in extremity leads. Because limits of normal were defined in the early days of electrocardiography before V leads were devised, the QRS duration is more satisfactorily compared with "normal" in the extremity leads.

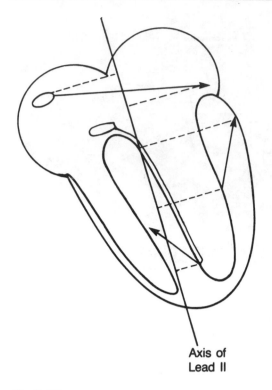

Axis of
Lead II

Fig. I–160

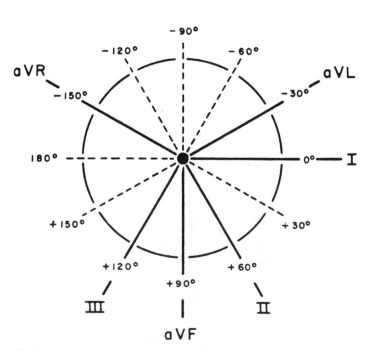

Fig. I–161

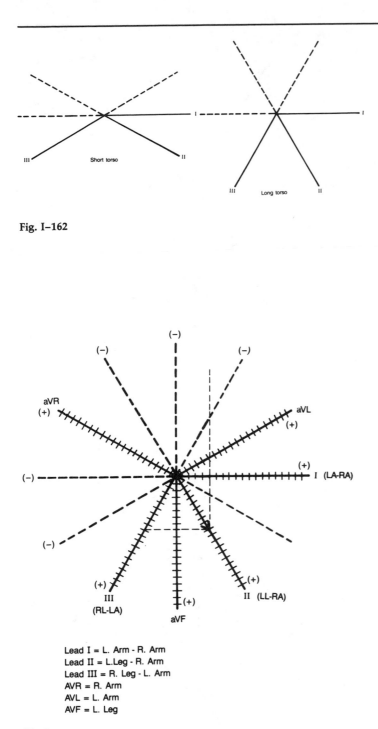

Fig. I–162

Lead I = L. Arm - R. Arm
Lead II = L.Leg - R. Arm
Lead III = R. Leg - L. Arm
AVR = R. Arm
AVL = L. Arm
AVF = L. Leg

Fig. I–163

EXTREMITY LEADS

The arrangement of the frontal plane leads is seen in Figure I–161. One must realize that few individuals are of such body build as to fit this scheme with the angles between extremity leads exactly as diagrammed; the 5-foot short-torso subject and the basketball player might differ as widely as shown in Figure I–162. Therefore, too much weight should not be given to a precise estimation of vector directions. Allowing for this obvious limitation, calculation of vector direction can be carried out as illustrated in Figure I–163.

If, for example, the QRS on lead I included a 5-mm upright R wave and a 1-mm negative S wave, the net projection of that QRS on lead I is +4. If the QRS on lead aVF includes a 1-mm Q wave plus a 6-mm R wave, the net projection on aVF is +5. Extending perpendiculars from 4 mm on lead I and 5 mm on aVF produces an intercept as shown. An arrow drawn from the 0 hub of the leads to this intercept indicates the direction and magnitude of the QRS force (net dipole). In this case, angles are calculated positively, clockwise from the positive (left) axis of lead I, and negatively, counterclockwise from the leftward axis of lead I.

Left-axis deviation *can* be defined simply by the net QRS deflection's being more downward than upward in lead II, whereas right-axis deviation can be recognized when the net QRS deflection is more downward than upward in lead I. The record with a predominantly downward QRS in both leads I and II does present a problem. What should this be called: severe left-axis deviation or severe right-axis deviation? It may be more useful to state that the net vector lies in the

180° to 270° quadrant (the positive extension of lead I being 0°).

When the net QRS is positive in aVL and negative in aVF and upright in lead II as seen in Figure I–164, the net vector lies between 0° and −30°. Some prefer to classify this as "horizontal heart position," reserving "left-axis deviation" for those records with a net vectoral direction more negative than −30°.

When the net projection is positive on aVF and slightly positive on lead I, "vertical" heart position may be recognized; whereas the combination of negative projection on lead I and positive projection on aVF would be classified as right-axis deviation (Fig. I–165).

As seen in Figure I–166, the V leads are arranged in a radical fashion. These leads do not lie in a simple horizontal (transverse) plane, but rather lie in a staircase fashion between V_2 and V_4 (see Fig. I–141).

To "construct" the V lead record, one may transfer the .01- to .02-sec dipole vector generated in the septum to the hub of the V leads and drop perpendiculars on the axes of each lead as shown in Figure I–166. This initial depolarization produces initial deflections, reflecting the projections of the dipole on each lead.

The .04- to .08-sec dipole vector is normally directed as shown in Figure I–166; it casts a large projection on many of the leads, being least powerfully represented on those leads lying most nearly at 90° to the .04 to .08 vector.

The .03 vector requires inclusion of the apical dipole as shown in Figure I–166. As the projection of .01- to .02-sec dipole decreases from V_1 to V_2 to V_3, the contribution of the .03 apical vector increases. One can

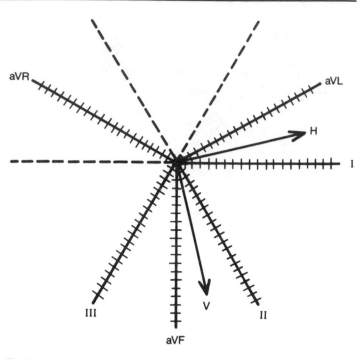

Fig. I–164

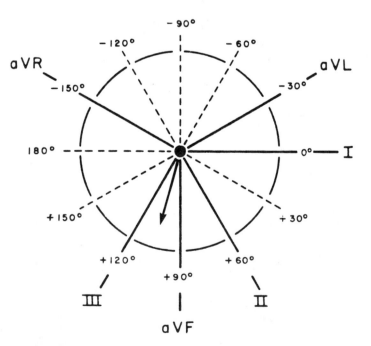

Fig. I–165

expect, in normal individuals, that R waves will grow taller from V_1 to V_6, S waves will grow smaller, and Q waves will appear in some left-sided leads. Because of the air-filled lung, however, voltage often dwindles from V_5 to V_6.

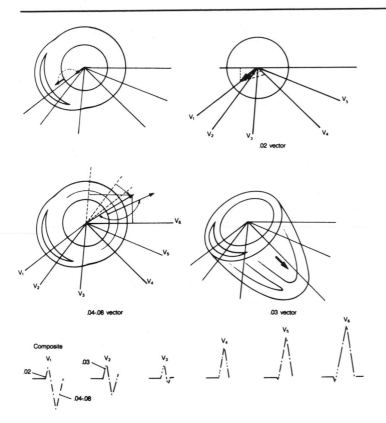

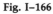

Fig. I–166

PART II

Interpretation of the Electrocardiogram

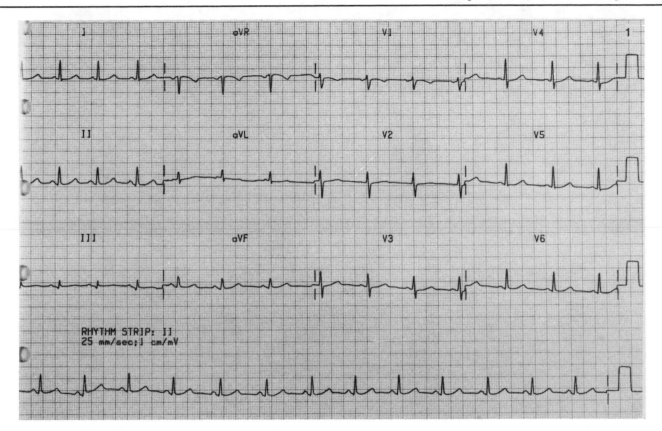

RHYTHM STRIP: II
25 mm/sec;1 cm/mV

EKG 1

This normal electrocardiogram is the product of the action potentials of a myriad of myocardial cells.

1. What is the action-potential duration of the representative cell in the ventricular myocardium?

ANSWER: The QRS complex begins with depolarization (phase 0) of the first cells to be activated. Normally, these cells lie on the left side of the ventricular septum. The T wave ends with completion of repolarization (phase 3) of the last cells to repolarize. They normally lie at the base of the free wall of the left ventricle. We know that the last cells to depolarize are those same basal free-wall cells, and we know their phase 0 occurs at the termination of the QRS complex. The action potential of those last cells thus extends from the final portion of the QRS (the J point) to the end of the T wave, in this case, 300 msec. Because these cells are representative of ventricular myocardial "working" cells, we may consider their action potentials to be fair modal samples of the ventricular population (remembering that a normal range of duration of action potential exists between short epicardial and longer subendocardial cells). Measure .300 sec on this EKG paper and remind yourself that these single-cell phenomena are large enough to be measured and are of a magnitude comparable to electrocardiographic time intervals. This helps relate the action potential to the EKG (see page 55).

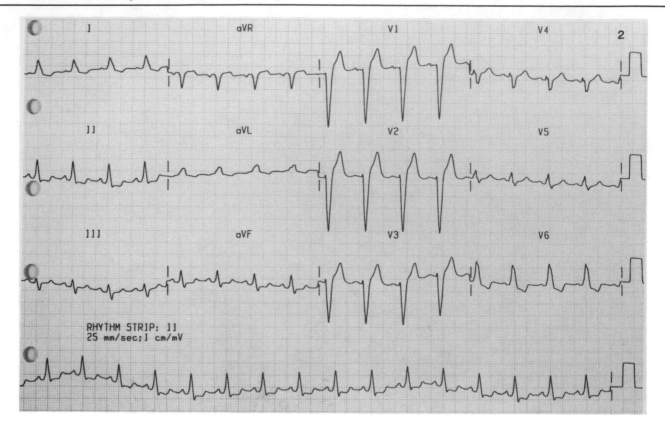

RHYTHM STRIP: 11
25 mm/sec;1 cm/mV

EKG 2

The most notable feature of this record is the wide QRS complex, indicating prolongation of intraventricular conduction time (.12 sec).

1. Where are the last ventricular cells to be depolarized?

ANSWER: The depolarizing dipole advances toward the pericardium, with its positive pole leading. The electrode that overlies the final advance of this dipole will register a terminal positive deflection (R wave). In this case, the last cells face the left side and thus lie on the left side of the heart.

2. Where are the first cells to depolarize?

ANSWER: Again, the advancing depolarizing dipole moves forward with a positive leading pole. Here, the first portion of the QRS is oriented toward the left. The septum must, therefore, be activated from right to left. This record indicates left bundle branch block. It is probably of the "washed-out bridge" variety. The lower branches of the left bundle system have probably survived, because the axis is not deviated to the left and the QRS duration is not greater than .12 sec.

3. Why are the T waves upright in leads V_1, V_2, and V_3 and inverted in lead V_6?

ANSWER: The first area to depolarize is the first to recover positive surface charge. Thus, the positive aspect of the repolarizing dipole faces the right in this situation in which depolarization and repolarization are delayed on the left.

4. Why are the S-T segments inclined upward on the right and downward on the left?

ANSWER: The S-T configuration here depends on the slope of phase 2 of the action potential. If that slope is a progressively steep one, indicating an accelerating accumulation of positive charge on the surface of the cells during phase 2 (and thus the S-T segment), the delay of electrical events in the region of the left bundle will result in an increasing disparity between the simultaneous positive surface charges of the cells of the blocked and unblocked region during phase 2. Right-side leads will register an upsloping and left-side leads a downsloping ST segment.

If phase 2 were horizontal, delay in depolarization and repolarization would not generate a difference in surface charge between the blocked and not blocked populations of cells and the S-T would remain isoelectric.

If, on the other hand, the rate of descent of phase 2 were constant, delay in intraventricular conduction would produce a constant difference in surface charge between blocked and unblocked populations of cells. The resulting S-T configuration would be horizontally elevated in leads recorded over the unblocked region and horizontally depressed in leads from the delayed zone.

To visualize this situation, draw an action potential with each of the three varieties of phase 2 mentioned. On a second piece of thin paper, overdraw the silhouette of each. Then displace the overlying paper slightly to the right to simulate a conduction delay and note the disparity in surface charges produced, reminding yourself that a downward deflection represents acquisition of positive surface charge.

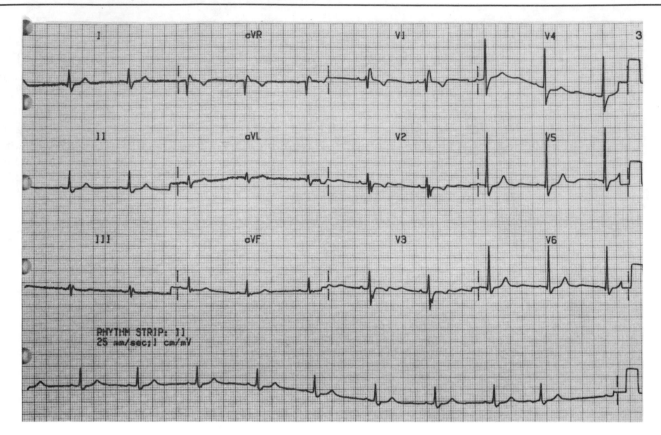

EKG 3

The QRS duration is prolonged in this record also.

1. Which direction do the final depolarizing dipoles face?

ANSWER: As seen in leads I, V_1, and V_6, they face to the right and anteriorly, producing a late R′ in V_1 and a negative S wave in leads I and V_6. Thus, the final enclave of cells to depolarize lies on the right.

2. Which direction do the first depolarizing dipoles face?

ANSWER: Again, leads V_1 and left-sided leads indicate a rightward orientation of these dipoles. Thus, the interventricular septum is activated in a normal left-to-right fashion.

3. If this represents right bundle branch block, why does the *thin* right ventricular free-wall so lag in depolarization as to exceed the time of depolarization of the much thicker left ventricular wall?

ANSWER: The right ventricular wall is depolarized lengthwise from apex to base in the absence of right bundle function. The "trip" for the dipole is thus much longer than the 3-mm thickness of the wall would suggest.

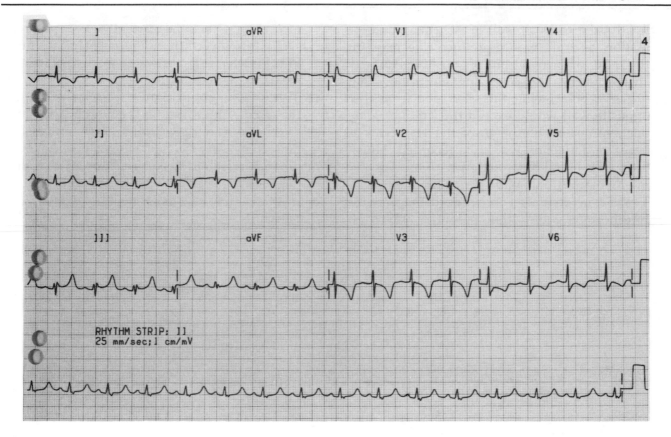

RHYTHM STRIP: II
25 mm/sec; 1 cm/mV

EKG 4

This record reveals right bundle branch block. Unlike the previous tracing, there are significant T-wave inversions in all V leads and in leads I, and aVL in this electrocardiogram. In the presence of bundle branch block, T waves are inverted over the area of delayed depolarization and are most severely inverted in V_1 in right bundle branch block and in V_5 and V_6 in left bundle branch block.

1. In this record with RBBB, the T-wave inversions are not deepest in the most rightward leads, but in the anterior and left lateral regions. What abnormality does this represent?

ANSWER: These symmetrically inverted T waves indicate a deficiency in positive surface charges during repolarization of the anterior and lateral ventricular walls.

2. What sort of deficiency?

ANSWER: Either (a) a loss of cells with loss of sarcolemmal surface upon which positive charge can be mounted in repolarization, or (b) a delay in repolarization as a result of prolongation of the action potential in the anterior and lateral region, or (c) abnormally rapid re-

polarization of the subendocardial cells of this region, generating a dipole with its negative pole facing the electrodes of leads V_2 through V_6 and leads I and aVL.

3. Why should the action potentials be shortened in the subendocardium?

ANSWER: Ischemia generally is progressively more severe as one advances from epicardium to endocardium, because obstruction of the "surface" coronary arteries is productive of increasing perfusion deficit in the more distal ramifications of the penetrating arteries. If ischemia in this instance has induced foreshortening of the action potential in proportion to the degree of ischemia, repolarization of the ischemic wall will advance from endo- to epicardium, with a negative leading pole.

4. But we stated in the preceding question and answer that the T waves here might reflect *prolongation* rather than *shortening* of the action potential. Can we have it both ways?

ANSWER: Both shortening and lengthening of the action potential by ischemia have been documented. Prolongation of action potential in a focal area as a result of ischemia, inflammation, or drugs would produce a decrease in the rate of generation of positive surface charge facing the overlying electrode. The negative pole facing this electrode from the opposite wall would exceed the simultaneous positive charge of the proximal wall, and a negative deflection would be recorded. Thus, focal transmural dysfunction with focal delay in repolarization may generate the same T-wave inversion as ischemic damage with foreshortening of action potential, which is most severe subendocardially and progressively less severe from endo- to epicardium.

5. What might be a reasonable expression of the meaning of this record?

ANSWER: One could report most literally that the record indicates a segmental abnormal "process." In our civilization, this "process" is most frequently ischemic; however, we should remind ourselves that *any* disorder that has depleted, delayed, or accelerated sarcolemmal repolarization can generate this type of abnormality.

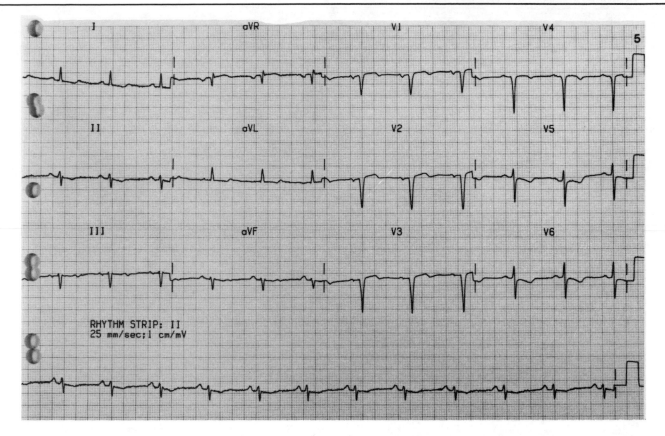

RHYTHM STRIP: II
25 mm/sec; 1 cm/mV

EKG 5

No R waves exist in leads V_1 through V_4 and only diminutive R waves occur in leads V_5 and V_6.

1. What is the meaning of this abnormality?

ANSWER: Depolarizing dipoles that normally advance toward these leads through the anterior septal and anterior myocardial walls are so depleted that those dipoles advancing through the normal posterior wall are not counter-balanced. As a result, the negative aspects of the posterior dipoles outnumber the positive poles of the anterior wall.

2. Have all the cells in an area been destroyed?

ANSWER: No, only enough that the cell population becomes less numerous than that of the opposite wall. Thus, the deeper is the QS, the more total is the destruction in the area.

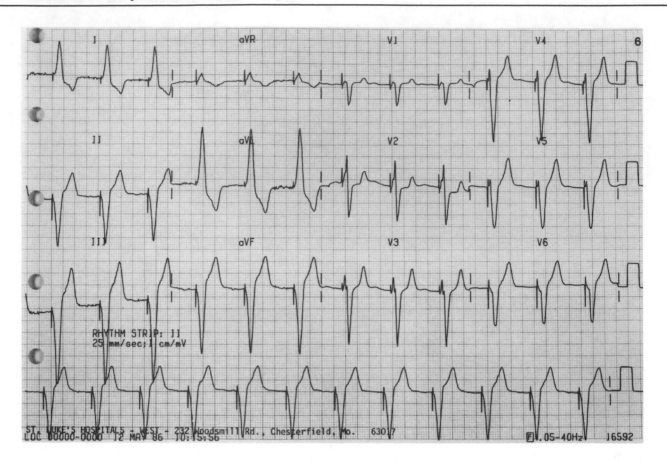

EKG 6

This is the record of an extrinsic ventricular pacemaker.

1. Where is the stimulating electrode?

ANSWER: Observe the QRS in three leads: an inferior lead (aVF), a lateral lead (I), and an anterior lead (V_1). Using these three leads and recognizing the fact that the depolarizing dipole creates an upright deflection when it advances toward an electrode and a negative deflection when it retreats from the electrode, aVF here indicates an inferior, lead I a rightward, and V_1 an anterior electrode position. By this "triangulation," the origin of the paced beats is identified in the anterior inferior portion of the right ventricle.

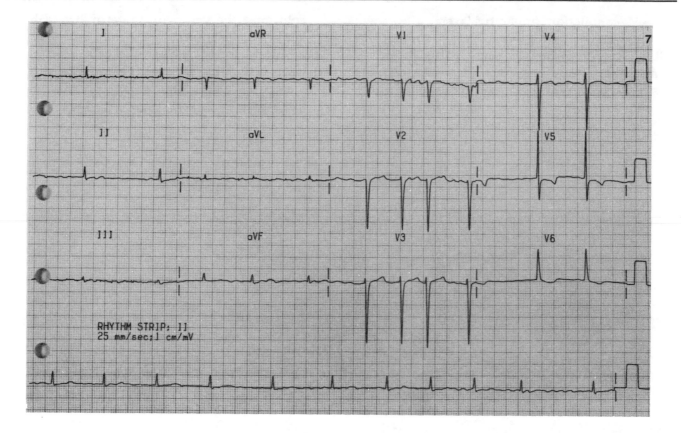

EKG 7

1. What is the atrial rhythm?

ANSWER: Atrial activity usually is studied best in lead V_1 because the examining electrode lies close to the atria in this lead. The constantly changing "wiggles" of the baseline indicate absence of an organized atrial depolarization; instead, they show a constantly fluctuating display of depolarization, atrial fibrillation.

2. If the refractory period of the A-V nodal tissue persists for 300 ± 100 msec after each conducted atrial beat, how can the interval between conducted beats in this record range from 440 to 720 msec?

ANSWER: If the broad-faced A-V node allows entry of a depolarization at one "portal," a second depolarization may enter another portal only to fall on the refractory tail of the first beat descending into the bundle of His (Case 7). This second beat may depolarize the upper portion of the node and thereby block entry of the third depolarization. Thus, two beats may be blocked by the "collisions"

within the "funnel" of the A-V node. Such concealed conduction and consequent block reduces the frequency of ventricular depolarization in atrial fibrillation and illustrates the importance of the anatomic shape of the A-V node.

3. If that is the case, what would result if the

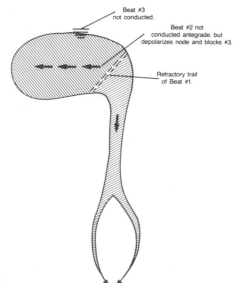

Case 7

A-V conduction apparatus were a narrow bridge rather than a broad faced "funnel"?

ANSWER: The answer is seen in the "experiment" of nature, the Wolff-Parkinson-White syndrome, in which "funnel" collisions do not occur in the slender accessory bridge. With no collisions, the ventricular rate in atrial fibrillation is determined by the refractory period of the accessory pathway. Thus, beats may occur at 200 to 300 msec intervals in Wolff-Parkinson-White syndrome during atrial fibrillation.

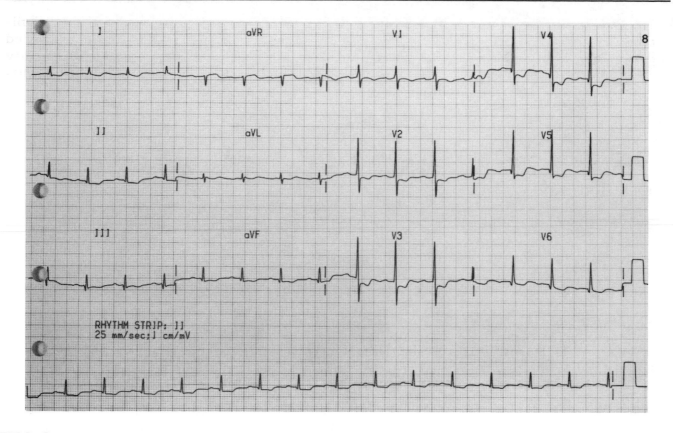

RHYTHM STRIP: II
25 mm/sec;1 cm/mV

EKG 8

The S-T segments are impressively depressed in V_2 to V_5, with depression throughout the S-T from onset (J point) to T wave.

1. What does this mean?

ANSWER: Total S-T depression in the absence of intraventricular conduction delay, especially if horizontal or downsloping, is seen when resting potential of an area of ventricular myocardium is subnormal, (Case 8). In this instance, the area of normal resting potential is sandwiched between the electrode and the damaged tissue. Thus, the lesion in this case may lie in the anterior subendocardium or in the posterior transmural region.

2. Does the QRS configuration indicate which of these alternatives is likely here?

ANSWER: The tall R waves in leads V_1 through V_3 are compatible with loss of posterior myocardium. The record is therefore compatible with an acute posterior infarction.

3. If this is an infarction, where are the "injured" cells with subnormal resting potential?

ANSWER: An infarct is not a block of total necrosis. Among the dead cells are many surviving hypoxic cells whose sarcolemmal pumps cannot so reposition sodium and potassium as to generate normal resting potential. Other so-injured cells lie around the "suburbs" of the infarction.

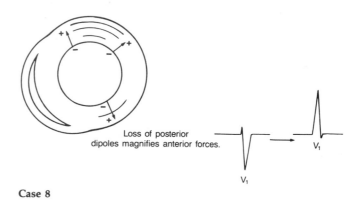

Loss of posterior
dipoles magnifies anterior forces.

V_1

V_1

Case 8

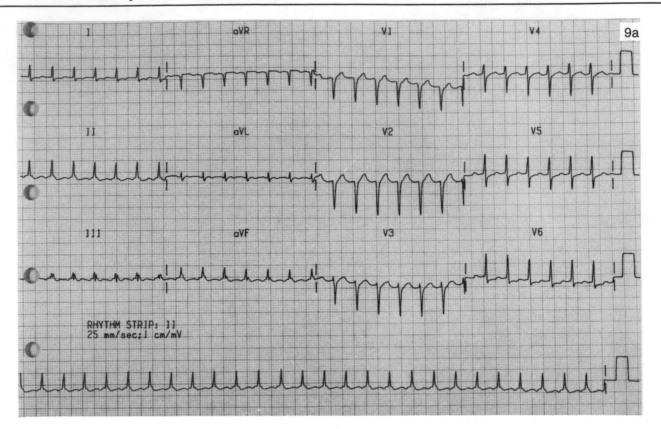

EKG 9

This rapid regular ventricular rhythm is supra-ventricular in origin.

1. What is the atrial rhythm?

ANSWER: The atrial rhythm can be determined best in lead aVF in record 9a. Often, atrial arrhythmias are best defined in aVF rather than in lead V_1. This may be because the long axis of the atrial depolarization path is projected well on a longitudinal lead (aVF). Note the inverted P waves occurring at twice the rate of the ventricular beats (320 vs. 160). The continual undulation of the baseline indicates no diastolic pause between atrial beats. This record therefore can be classified atrial flutter with 2:1 A-V block.

Record 9b followed electrical cardioversion.

2. What is the rhythm?

ANSWER: It is normal sinus rhythm with a rare atrial premature contraction.

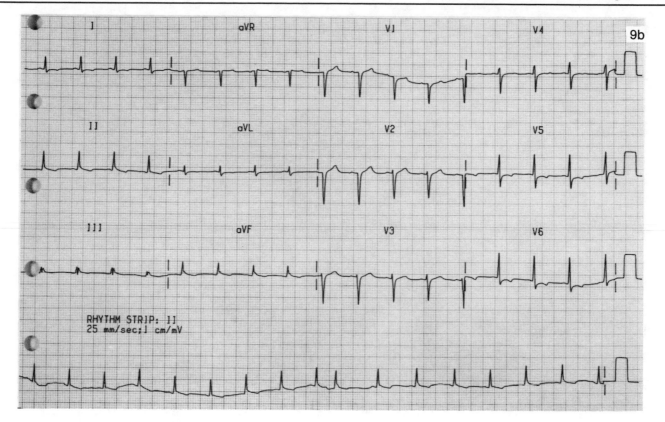

I   aVR   V1   V4   9b

II   aVL   V2   V5

III   aVF   V3   V6

RHYTHM STRIP: II
25 mm/sec;1 cm/mV

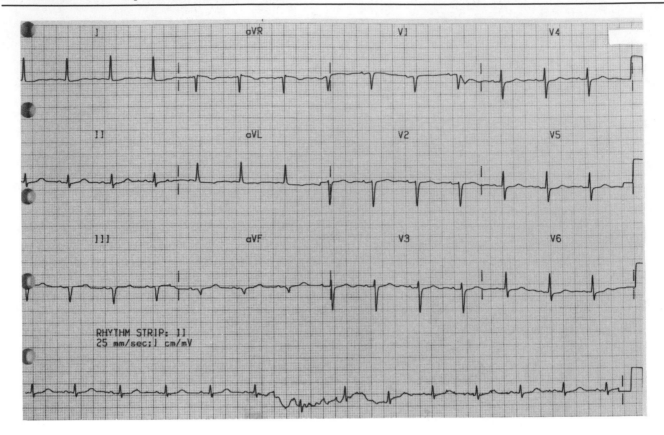

EKG 10

1. What is the significance of the QS in lead aVF and in lead III?

ANSWER: The normal R wave in aVF occurs within .03 sec after onset of the QRS complex (see page 10) as the inferior wall is depolarized in a footward direction. Loss of this R wave indicates either (a) loss of sarcolemmal depolarization in the diaphragmatic wall or (b) abnormal direction of depolarization, for example, as in some instances of left bundle branch block in which depolarization is directed from right to left and from apex toward base. In that situation, the QS in lead aVF occurs in association with prolongation of QRS in the configuration of LBBB and does not pose a difficult problem for interpretation. Loss of sarcolemmal depolarization is most commonly a result, in Western society, of is-

chemic myocardial infarction. It must be remembered, however, that other causes of sarcolemmal nonfunction—traumatic damage, inflammatory process, and tumors—on occasion produce focal loss of cell function with generation of pathologic Q waves or QS configurations. Nonetheless, infarction is most likely here.

2. Does the QS in lead III have the significance of the QS in aVF?

ANSWER: No. Lead III lies in such a direction as to produce large Q waves or QS complexes in some normal persons (see page 57). It is a good rule to "test" the apparent abnormality seen in lead III by the configuration of other leads, especially aVF and lead II. In fact, if it were not a traditional component of the 12-lead system, lead III might be discarded because it adds no reliable data to the other 11 leads.

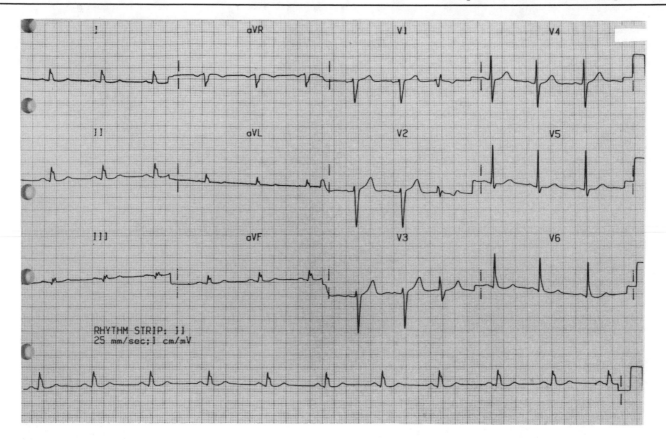

RHYTHM STRIP: II
25 mm/sec; 1 cm/mV

EKG 11

The QRS duration of .10 indicates an intra-ventricular conduction delay here. The terminal QRS deflections in left-sided leads indicate the delay is on the left, because final depolarization dipoles are facing (advancing toward) the left.

1. Does this represent a form of left bundle branch block?

ANSWER: The initial Q waves in leads I, II, III, aVF, V_5 and V_6 give the answer. They indicate that initial (septal) depolarization is directed from the left toward the right. The left side of the septum is depolarized "on time." The interventricular conduction delay seen here,

therefore, is not a result of left bundle branch block (as seen earlier, LBBB abolishes the normal left-sided Q waves generated in the septum). Nor is the delay a result of RBBB, because no RR^1 exists in lead V_1 and no S in leads I, V_5, and V_6. The delay is *distal* to the bundles. It may be a result of conduction delay through the free wall of the left ventricular because of damage in that area or it may be the result of an increase in mass of the left ventricular myocardium. One might classify this record as peripheral interventricular conduction delay.

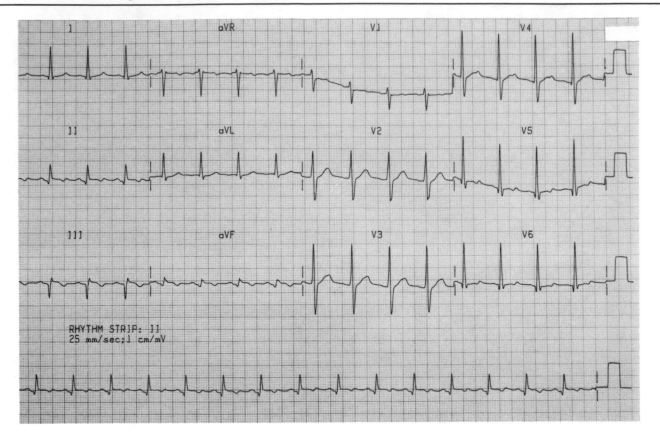

EKG 12

The Q wave in lead aVF is .04 sec in duration.
1. Is this normal?

ANSWER: No. The upper limit of normal of Q-wave duration is .02 to .03 sec, as was discussed on page 10. This Q wave indicates loss of depolarizing dipoles in the inferior left ventricular wall. Unlike the QS in lead aVF in EKG 10, this lead aVF presents the pathologic Q wave followed by a stubby, broad R wave, and a prolonged QRS (QRS=.10 sec). What does this mean? The QR complex seen here, with .04-sec Q wave does indicate loss of sarcolemmal activity (usually the result of ischemic cell necrosis); however, the R wave indicates survival of cells in the more superficial layers of the depolarization myocardial wall. Those cells are delayed in their depo-

larization by the obstruction of conduction through the necrotic subendocardial and mid-myocardial strata. The depolarizing process may be considered as "picking its way" through slowly conducting and round-about pathways through the damaged area. The configuration seen in aVF should be interpreted as diaphragmatic infarction with peri-infarction block.

2. Is this purely a subendocardial infarction?

ANSWER: No, if subendocardial infarction denotes an infarction that does not produce a pathologic Q wave because only the self-cancelling subendocardial 3 to 4 mm of myocardium are necrotic. This lesion extends farther into the middle strata and has produced a Q wave because of loss of those middle layer cells that normally depolarize at .04 sec.

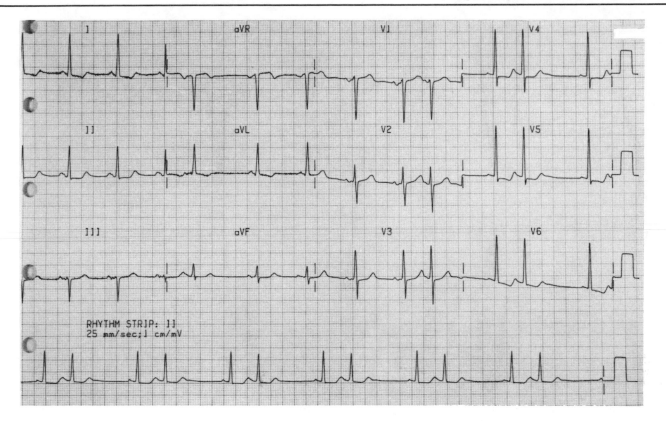

RHYTHM STRIP: II
25 mm/sec; 1 cm/mV

EKG 13

Among the striking features of this record are the increase in QRS voltage and the S-T,T configuration.

1. Could this be a normal variant?

ANSWER: No, even normal children or thin adults whose tissues conduct electricity to the body surface so easily as to produce high-voltage QRS complexes would not generate the features seen here. (In children, the sum of S-wave depth in V_1 and R-wave height in V_5 or V_6 may normally reach 45 mm; whereas in normal adults, these amounts rarely exceed 35 mm.) The downsloping S-T and diphasic or downward T in leads I, aVL, and V_4 through V_6, and the deep S in V_1, and tall R in V_5 and V_6 comprise three of the four changes generated by left ventricular hypertrophy (the fourth characteristic not seen here is QRS prolongation, as discussed on page 14). Another indicator of left ventricular enlargement is increased height of the R wave in lead aVL. The R wave in this lead, which "faces" the free

wall of the left ventricle in many instances, normally does not exceed 11 mm.

2. What is the importance of the P wave notching and prolongation in this record?

ANSWER: The normal duration of the P wave (.10 sec) represents the time required for the depolarization process to march across the atria from the right upper region of the right atrium to the left wall of the left atrium. Left atrial enlargement lengthens this journey and is frequently manifested by prolongation of the P wave. The second half of the P wave is formed by the left atrium. When the left atrium is dilated, the second portion of the P wave is enlarged. This enlargement follows the normal "dimple" or notch at the midpoint, ascribed by some to normal deflection of depolarization into the interatrial septum. This record reveals prolongation and enlargement of the second portion of the P wave, indicative of left atrial enlargement. Because the "peripheral resistance" of the left atrium is the mitral valve and the left ventricle, left atrial enlargement, in the absence of mitral disease, implies loss of left ventricular compliance and suggests myocardiopathy, hypertrophy, or dilatation.

3. What does the diphasic P wave in lead V_1 indicate?

ANSWER: The electrode position in V_1 and/or V_2 sits astride the atria with a "50-yard-line seat." As the dipole advances across the right atrium, it generates a positive deflection in the first half of the P wave. As it moves past the "reviewing stand" of the electrode, its negative trailing edge is produced by left atrial depolarization. Thus, V_1 and/or V_2 provides a means of recognizing right and left atrial states. When the left atrium is dilated, the negative second half of the P wave often is longer than .045 sec and deeper than 1 mm.

4. Does the diphasic configuration of P wave alone denote an abnormality?

ANSWER: No, it merely locates the position of the electrode at the midpoint between right and left atrial walls. Disease is indicated by excessive *duration* or *amplitude* of a component of the P wave.

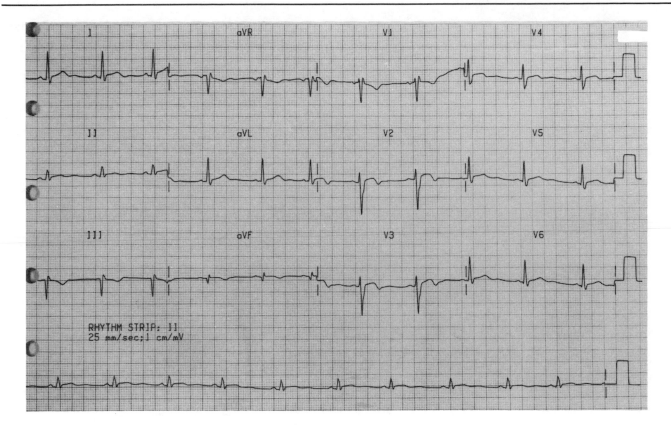

RHYTHM STRIP: II
25 mm/sec; 1 cm/mV

EKG 14

QRS duration here is .10 to .11 sec; RR' occurs in V_1, and there are S waves in leads I, V_5 and V_6, and normal Q waves in leads I, aVL, V_5, and V_6.

1. What conduction abnormality is this?

ANSWER: The delayed depolarization process faces rightward. The initial septal depolarization proceeds from left to right. The record represents a conduction defect that impedes the arrival of dipoles in the right and anterior portion of the heart. As described on page 20, this delay in activation of the right ventricle most frequently is a result of right bundle branch block. As indicated on page 22, other conditions that may prolong the process of depolarization from the apex to the base of the right ventricular wall are (a) right ventricular dilatation and (b) congenital foreshortening of the right bundle. In the latter case, the conduction delay is usually minimal, with QRS duration often ranging from .08 to .10 sec. In fact, this condition in a small, normal-sized heart may produce the RR' in leads V_1, and S in leads I and V_5 and V_6 without extension of QRS duration beyond the usual limits of normal. Such individuals, if they did not have a shortened right bundle, might have a QRS duration of .05, .06, and .07 sec. In them, QRS duration of .07, .08, and .09 sec represents a prolongation.

2. Why are T waves inverted in leads V_1 through V_3?

ANSWER: The last area to be depolarized is also the last to be repolarized. Therefore, during T-wave inscription, the surface charge on the cells of the right side of the septum and the right ventricular wall are less positive at each instant than normal. The resulting difference in simultaneous surface charge creates the negative T wave in leads recorded over the right ventricle. For the same reasons, the T wave is inverted in leads V_5 and V_6 that overlie an area of delayed depolarization in the presence of left bundle branch block and left ventricular hypertrophy.

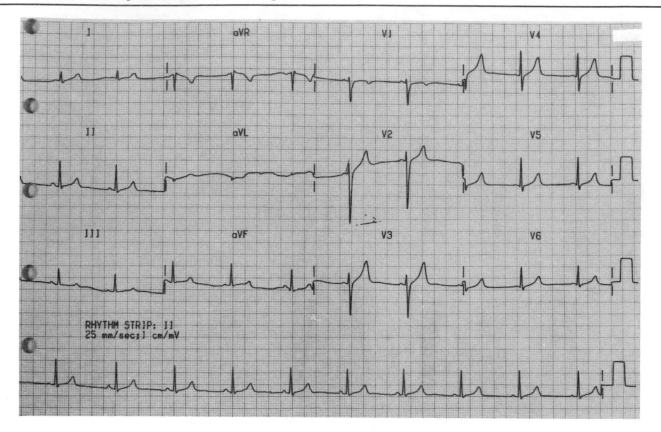

EKG 15

In this record, the T waves are tall or peaked.

1. What is the mechanism?

ANSWER: Because the T wave is the composite of the phase 3 of a myriad of myocardial cells and is generated by differences in simultaneous surface charges, the normal variations in the steepness of phase 3 are reflected in variations in the height of the normal T wave. When phase 3 in all cells is steep, the difference between a representative early cell's repolarization and a late cell's repolarization is great; whereas a normal cell population with a more gentle, sloping phase 3 would produce a smaller difference in potential and a less peaked T wave.

2. What electrolyte disorder might produce such tall T waves?

ANSWER: In the presence of hyperkalemia, phase 3 becomes much more steep (one can reason in childlike fashion that if there is more of something, its action will take place more rapidly (at least this is a memory aid), and as a result, the T wave becomes tall and pointed.

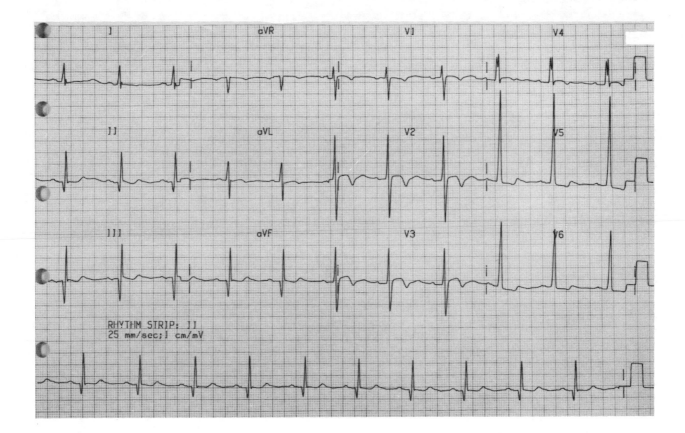

EKG 16

Note the Q waves in leads II, III, and aVF; the T waves in leads V_1 through V_4; the S-T,T configuration in V_5 and V_6; and the tall R waves in V_5 and V_6. This is a complex record.

1. What is the meaning of the QR in leads II, III, and aVF?

ANSWER: These are pathologic Q waves because they are .04 sec in duration. This is the essential feature of the abnormal Q wave, because it means the dipoles that normally generate R waves after .03 sec are not present. This is the result of sarcolemmal loss as in infarction. As we pointed out elsewhere, the Q-R complex indicates the survival of cells in or near the area of infarction.

2. The T waves become deeper from V_1 to V_2, then less deep in V_3. Can this be normal?

ANSWER: No. T waves may normally be inverted in V_1 and V_2 because the apical area may repolarize so as to present negative aspects of the dipoles to the right. However, the normal T wave becomes less inverted as one progresses from V_1 to V_2 and 3_3. Whenever the T wave becomes deeper as one moves from V_1 to V_2 to V_3, an abnormality is present. When, as in this case, the deepest T wave is localized, with less deep or upright T waves in neighboring leads, the dipole deficit is localized. In this case, the loss of repolarizing dipoles lies in the anteroseptal area. As was discussed earlier, this is most frequently an ischemic process.

The tall R waves and S-T,T in leads V_5 and V_6 and the broad notched P waves indicate left ventricular hypertrophy and left atrial enlargement.

Thus, this patient has had a diaphragmatic infarction and anteroseptal damage in the presence of left ventricular hypertrophy and left atrial enlargement.

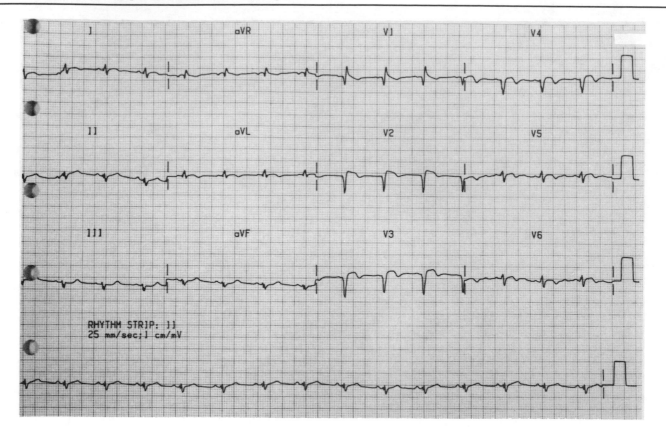

RHYTHM STRIP: II
25 mm/sec; 1 cm/mV

EKG 17

This electrocardiogram reveals an anteroseptal anterior infarction.

1. What is the meaning of the QR in lead V_1?

ANSWER: It indicates dipoles advancing anteriorly toward the right late in the ventricular depolarization period. This wave may be moving toward the base of the ventricles through the septum or through the free wall of the right ventricle.

Its delayed occurrence indicates either peri-infarction conduction delay in the septum or delay in the right ventricle. In either case, S waves would be seen in leads I, V_5 and V_6.

2. The S-T segments are elevated in leads V_2 through V_5. Does this indicate acute myocardial injury?

ANSWER: Two possibilities exist: the elevations may reflect the acute cellular injury associated with a recent infarction, or they may reflect the stretching of sarcolemma produced by aneurysmal deformity of an old infarction.

3. The voltage is low. This may represent pericardial effusion. What else might lower the voltage in this situation?

ANSWER: Loss of myocardial cells may reduce the voltage. Voltage may be diminished in the presence of normal myocardial cell population when poorly conductive tissue is interposed between the heart and the body surface. Because both air and fat conduct electricity poorly, emphysema and obesity are common causes of a loss of voltage. This record, therefore, may be that of a patient with infarct whose myocardial cell population is widely depleted or that of a patient with infarction complicated by pericardial effusion, emphysema, or obesity.

4. Can *focal* myocardial damage as seen in infarction reduce voltage?

ANSWER: Loss of myocardium in a limited area produces QS or QR configuration in overlying leads and abnormally *tall* R waves in opposite leads, but voltage decreases only when dipole force is reduced in many directions. Thus, widespread myocardial cell loss is implied when voltage loss results from myocardial damage. Myocardial disease without loss of cells may be manifested by loss of voltage when a diffuse process infiltrates the interstitium with such less-conductive matter as amyloid or the mucoprotein of myxedema.

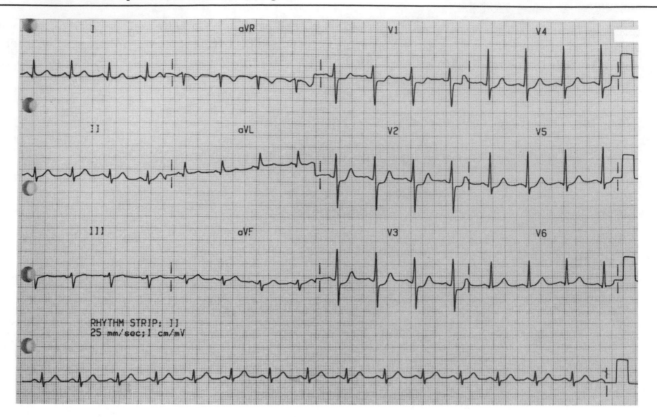

EKG 18

S-T segments are depressed in leads V_1 through V_4.

1. What is the significance of the fact that the *entire* S-T segment from J point to T wave is depressed?

ANSWER: Depression or elevation of the latter portion of the S-T segment reflects deformity of the second half of phase 2 of the action potential and is often the result of digitalis effect, left ventricular strain, or sympatho-mimetic activity. Horizontal depression or elevation of the whole S-T segment may result from sarcolemmal dysfunction so severe that the resting potential of cells in the damaged region of the myocardium is reduced. Horizontal S-T elevation or depression also may reflect such severe sarcolemmal damage that the entire length of phase 2 of the action potential is deformed. This record, therefore, indicates severe sarcolemmal damage.

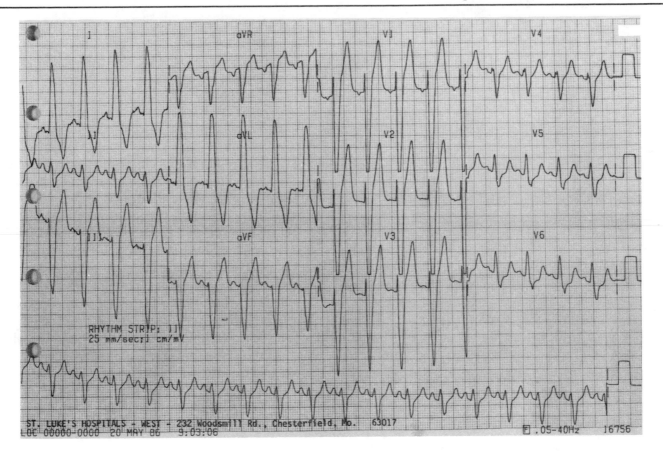

EKG 19

A marked intraventricular conduction delay (QRS .15 sec) with increased voltage and small Q waves in leads I and aVL are seen. The S-T segment is horizontally depressed in leads V_5 and V_6. S waves are prominent in leads II, III, aVF, and V_1 through V_6, and left axis deviation exists.

1. Can all of these features be attributed to LBBB?

ANSWER: In LBBB, when the lower portion of the left bundle system does not conduct, depolarization introduced by way of the right bundle advances in oblique circumferential fashion around the left ventricle from apex to base, with the negative aspect of the dipoles facing the inferior anteroseptal and anterior leads during left ventricular depolarization.

In this case, the *greatly* increased voltage suggests the additional presence of left ventricular enlargement. (LBBB may increase voltage because all dipoles may "face the same direction" and the normal partial cancellation produced by simultaneous depolarization of opposite walls does not occur. The precise limits of voltage increase resulting from LBBB are debatable; however, the voltage seen here exceeds that produced by LBBB.)

2. How can Q waves occur in left-sided leads I and aVL in LBBB?

ANSWER: One may be more comfortable if one assumes this large heart (left ventricular hypertrophy) lies in a horizontal position, with the apex pointing leftward. Thus, depolarization of the septum through the right bundle may advance not only right-to-left but also *apex-to-base*, generating negative impact on some left-sided leads even in LBBB. The S waves in leads V_4 through V_6 are in part the result of the same factor, with free-wall depolarization advancing from apex (left) to base (rightward).

The S-T depressions in leads V_5 and V_6 resemble the horizontal depressions attributed to myocardial injury.

3. Must acute injury be added to the list of this patient's cardiac problems?

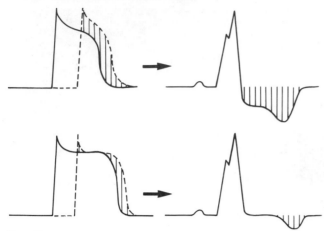

Case 19

ANSWER: Maybe. It is possible that this represents the same damage as that discussed on pages 28 through 35. Only serial records and perhaps tests for enzymes and other clinical data will tell; however, this horizontal S-T depression may be the result of LBBB alone.

If there is a significant delay between the first and last ventricular action potentials owing to LBBB or LVH, or both, the two-cell model of the situation may be as shown in Case 19.

If, by chance, phase 2 of the action potential were flat rather than sloping, the interventricular conduction delay would generate *no* S-T deviation:

Let us state these important facts again: the slope of phase 2, which *normally* may be *flat* or *sloping,* determines the isoelectric or depressed S-T configuration when intraventricular conduction is delayed. As illustrated in Case 19, it also influences the shape of the T wave. The greater the delay, the more marked the S-T and T changes can be. The patient with LBBB or LVH with S-T depressions suggestive of injury and T waves compatible with ischemia must be evaluated by serial records and clinical data before the presence or absence of an ischemic myocardium can be established.

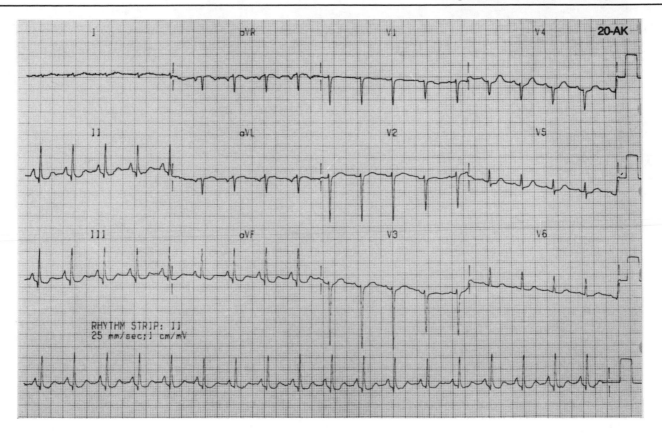

RHYTHM STRIP: II
25 mm/sec;1 cm/mV

EKG 20

1. What are some of the notable features here?

ANSWER: (a) The tall, peaked, "Christmas tree" P waves are indicative of right atrial enlargement (page 92).

(b) Vertical electrical position with an axis of $+90°$ and small R waves in leads V_1 through V_4 (clockwise rotation) may be generated by hyperinflation of the lungs and depression of the diaphragm, with resultant rotation of the heart to the left (clockwise). These findings may be produced by pulmonary disease with or without right ventricular enlargement. With P-wave evidence of right atrial enlargement as in this record, however, right ventricular hypertrophy can be assumed with confidence. Other manifestations of right ventricular hypertrophy are discussed elsewhere.

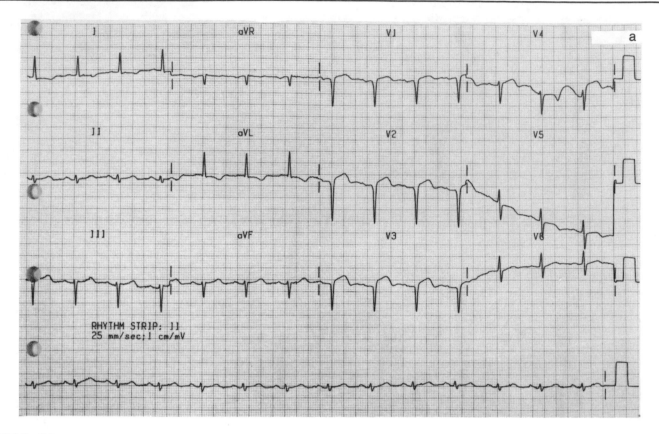

EKG 21

Record 21a was recorded immediately after the patient's admission to the hospital with acute anteroseptal anterior infarction. Record 21b was made a few days later. Both records show QS and S-T features indicative of acute infarction.

1. Explain the upsloping S-T segments and upright T waves in leads V_1 through V_3 in a and the inverted T waves in these leads in b.

ANSWER: The subnormal resting potential of the severely injured cells within the infarction would generate the illusion of horizontal elevation of the entire S-T segment in leads V_1 through V_3. The *upsloping* angle of the S-T segment requires an additional explanation: The accelerated repolarization of ischemic cells, manifested by a downsloping phase 2 and a shortened action potential, would create abnormally rapid acquisition of positive surface charges on these cells. As a result, the positive charges of the anteroseptal dipoles facing the electrodes V_1, V_2, V_3, and V_4 exceed the simultaneously generated negative charges facing the electrodes from the normal posterior wall. Because the excess positive charges would increase from beginning to the end of phase 2 and phase 3, the S-T segment would incline upward and the T wave would be positive in leads V_1, V_2, and V_3.

As the severely damaged cells die or recover, the ST elevation that resulted from the abnormality of their resting potential diminishes. In the course of uncomplicated acute infarction, T waves recorded over the lesion become inverted, as seen in Case 21. More than one factor plays a role in this "evolutionary" sequence: Acutely damaged but surviving cells may generate abnormally short action potentials, as has been mentioned, with premature acquisition of positive surface charges. The prematurity of repolarizing dipole generation matches the dipole deficit caused by depopulation. As the ischemic cells recover, the rate of their repolarization returns toward normal and accelerated repolarization no longer obscures the true loss of repolarization from cell death. A second factor contributes to the progressive T-in-T inversion seen in "evolution"

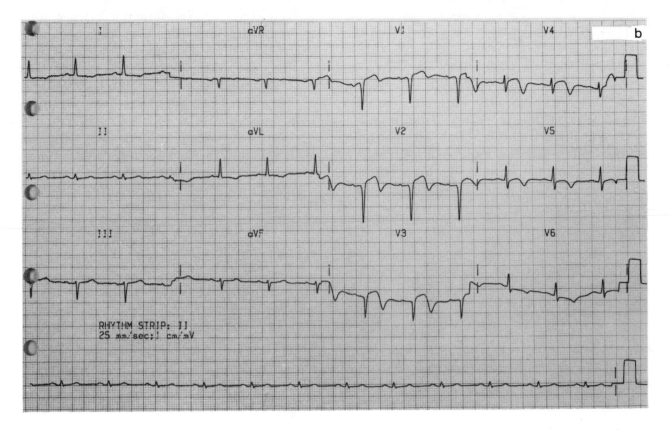

of the infarction. During the height of the initial event, the T wave may be "invisible" because it is incorporated in the downslope of the ST segment. As noted in EKG 21a, the T wave at that time is *in fact* negative because at each moment it lies below the true zero baseline that lies at the level of the S-T segment. As seen in EKG 21b, as this true baseline falls, the true relation of the T wave to the baseline becomes increasingly apparent. Thus, the classic "evolutionary" sequences with simultaneously falling S-T segment and T waves are to be expected.

The early T-wave behavior in this patient brings to mind the "hyperacute" T wave often seen in the first few minutes of infarction. That T-wave configuration, however, differs from that seen in EKG 21 in that the hyperacute T wave is a sharply peaked, tall T wave recorded by electrodes placed over the lesion.

2. Is there an additional explanation for the hyperacute T wave other than the ischemic shortening of action potential already mentioned?

ANSWER: Yes. The ischemic damage to the myocardium may also affect the intramyocardial sympathetic nerve endings, causing release of catecholamines, with a resulting shortening of the action potential.

3. If the ischemic lesion were transmural, would the initial T wave be abnormally tall as seen in this record?

ANSWER: Yes.

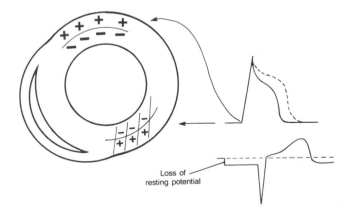

Loss of resting potential

Case 21

4. If the lesion were subendocardial, would the early change in the T wave be as described in this section?

ANSWER: No. Early repolarization as a direct effect of ischemia on myocardial cells or on sympathetic nerve endings, when limited to the inner layers of the myocardial wall, would produce a reverse of the normal sequence of repolarization, and the inner cells would repolarize before the normal, more superficial cells. The dipole so generated would produce negative T waves in the overlying leads.

5. Later, when ischemic cells die in the subendocardium, what would the T-wave configuration become?

ANSWER: The loss of inner layer cells in the adjacent wall would leave the negative dipole of the opposite wall uncancelled. Therefore, the terminal portion of the T wave generated by subendocardial cell loss is inverted. The degree of terminal T-wave inversion is proportional to the mass of cells lost in the inner layers. The early portion of the T wave remains upright in proportion to the degree of survival of the more superficial layers.

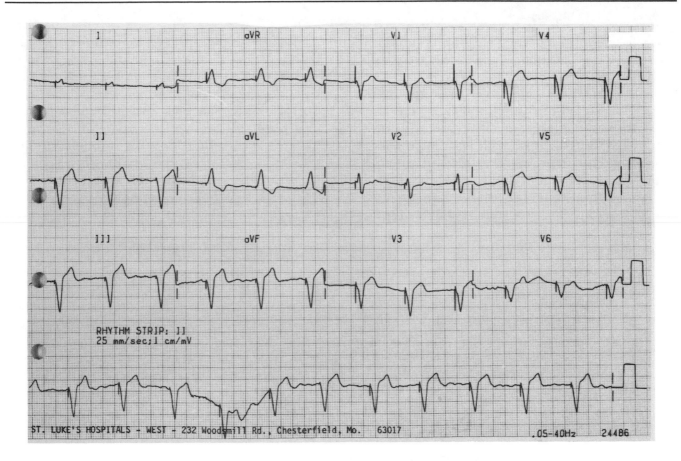

RHYTHM STRIP: II
25 mm/sec; 1 cm/mV

ST. LUKE'S HOSPITALS - WEST - 232 Woodsmill Rd., Chesterfield, Mo. 63017   .05-40Hz   24486

EKG 22

An extrinsic pacemaker is generating ventricular rhythm in the presence of atrial fibrillation.

1. Where is the stimulating electrode?

ANSWER: The QRS configuration in leads aVF, I, aVL, and V_1 permits precise "triangulation." In lead aVF, the predominant depolarization is moving away from the inferior myocardium; thus, the electrode lies in the inferior region. The small, but upright QRS in lead I and the upright QRS in lead aVL indicate rightward and cranial direction of dipole movement from the point of stimulation; thus, the electrode lies to the right and inferiorly. QRS in lead V_1 is predominantly negative, indicating posterior migration of the depolarizing process. The electrode therefore lies (1) inferiorly, (2) rightward, and (3) anteriorly. The common location for a transvenous pacemaker electrode is in the right ventricle, as seen here.

2. If that is the case, how do you explain the QS in leads V_5 and V_6?

ANSWER: This illustrates that the apex of the right ventricle lies at or near the cardiac apex. Indeed, chest roentgenograms of patients with transvenous pacemakers regularly show the electrode tip near the left border of the heart at its apex. The depolarizing dipole, therefore, moves rightward and upward from its origin.

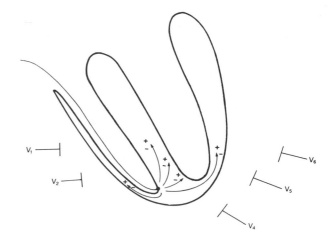

Case 22

Some of these leads present a small initial R wave following the pacemaker blip, followed by a large S wave (in lead V_1 for example).

3.   What does this mean?

ANSWER: This is the dipole generated in the wall interspaced between the pacemaker electrode and the recording electrode.

Note in this case the initial R wave is prominent in leads V_1 and V_2 and very small to absent in leads V_3 through V_6.

4.   How can this be?

ANSWER: (a) The depolarizing wave advances toward leads V_1 and V_2 through the overlying wall and septum. Its advance up the septum and free wall is directed away from leads V_5 and V_6. Later, the depolarizing wave marches up the free left-ventricular wall (Case 22).

(b) There has been loss of myocardium as a result of disease (i.e., infarction) between the electrode and leads V_3 through V_6. This finding would require review of pre-pacing records or examination of spontaneous ventricular beats when demand pacemaker action is suppressed.

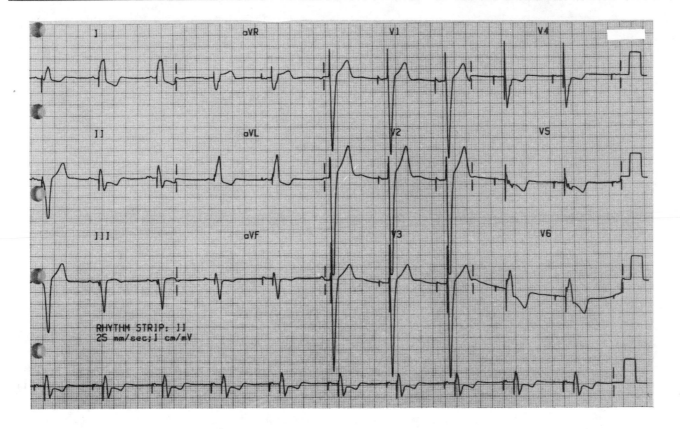

RHYTHM STRIP: II
25 mm/sec; 1 cm/mV

EKG 23

This is a more complex pacemaker record.

1. What type of pacemaker is this?

ANSWER: In one portion of the record, blips appear before the broad QRS complex, indicating ventricular stimulation. These blips and QRS complexes are preceded by P waves with consistent P-R intervals.

In another portion of the record, there are two blips, one preceding the P wave, one preceding the QRS complex. The blip-blip interval is constant.

This record is that of an A-V sequential pacemaker that is programmed to stimulate the atria when atrial rate is less than 59 to 60 beats per minute. The ventricular pacemaker is programmed to fire .16 sec after either a normal sinus beat or an atrial stimulus unless suppressed by ventricular depolarization.

The voltage is greater than normal and the QRS-T complexes in some ways suggest left ventricular hypertrophy.

2. Does this positively indicate left ventricular hypertrophy?

ANSWER: As in LBBB, right ventricular pacing produces depolarization in one general direction, with little or no cancellation of electrical forces going in opposite directions. Voltage in paced rhythms, therefore, may be magnified.

The S-T,T configurations in leads V_4 through V_6 are strikingly abnormal.

3. Is this related to the pacing?

ANSWER: Yes. The left wall of this heart is depolarized last and therefore repolarizes last. Thus, as in left bundle branch block and left ventricular hypertrophy, the S-T,T configuration in right ventricular paced rhythms reflects this sequence.

4. Can one recognize acute ischemic injury in a patient with a pacemaker?

ANSWER: If earlier records exist for comparison, marked S-T,T changes may raise suspicion of an active process.

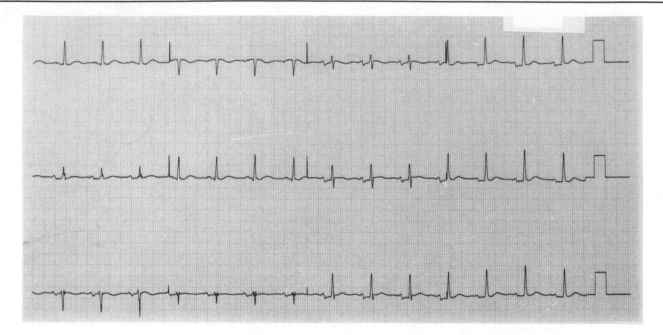

EKG 24

The Q-T interval ranges from .28 to .34 sec at a rate of 82 beats per minute. The S-T segment is notably *short* and downsloping in many leads.

1. What clinical possibilities come to mind?

ANSWER: Short Q-T intervals with a downsloping S-T segment over left-sided leads is most commonly the result of the action of digitalis or sympathomimetic drugs, or hyperactivity of the sympathetic nervous system.

2. This patient had received no such drugs. What else may produce these configurations?

ANSWER: Hypercalcemia. In fact, this patient had consumed 100 calcium-containing antacid tablets and at the time of this recording, serum calcium concentration was 15 mEq/L. This type of electrocardiogram may be helpful in other clinical settings; i.e., the problem of an unconscious patient with sluggish tendon jerks may be suspected from the electrocardiogram before the blood chemistry lab reports the calcium concentration. The important fact is that the patient is not receiving digitalis or sympathomimetic agents. In this day of illegal "street" drugs, we must remember the possibility of cocaine use in patients with this short, downsloping S-T configuration.

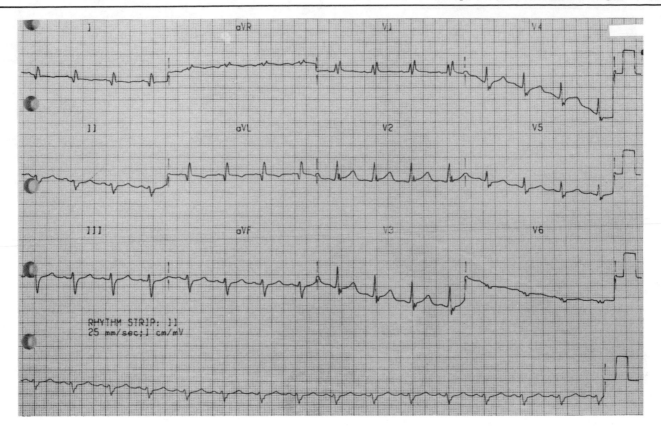

RHYTHM STRIP: II
25 mm/sec;1 cm/mV

EKG 25

This record represents intraventricular conduction delay with features indicative of right bundle branch block and left anterior hemiblock. In addition, there are .04-sec Q waves in lead I, .035-sec Q waves in lead aVL, and a notched QS in lead V_6.

1. How do you account for these latter findings?

ANSWER: Lateral myocardium has been lost, presumably as a result of infarction.

In right bundle branch block, one expects a prominent S wave in lead I.

2. Why is the S wave in lead I diminutive?

ANSWER: The left anterior hemiblock may be compounded by further peri-infarction conduction delay in the lateral wall of the left ventricle. As a result, the delay in conduction to the left partially cancels the effect of the delayed conduction through the free wall of the right ventricle produced by right bundle branch block.

3. Do other conditions exist in which one might see unusually small S waves in left-sided leads in the presence of right bundle branch block?

ANSWER: Any condition in which conduction into the free wall of the left ventricle is prolonged would generate this situation, provided delayed free-wall depolarization advances in a leftward direction.

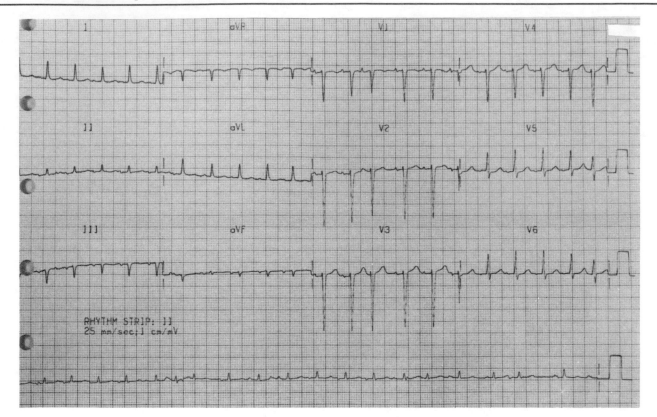

EKG 26

Note the P waves in this record.
1. What can you say about the location of the atrial pacemaker?

ANSWER: The inverted P waves in leads II, III, and aVF indicate a caudal location of the atrial pacemaker, while the normal P-R interval indicates its location above the A-V node. This has sometimes been designated as coronary sinus rhythm because the orifice of the coronary sinus lies in the atrium just above the A-V node.

The P waves in this record vary in configuration and the P-R interval varies from .12 to .19 sec. The variation in configuration and P-R interval is appreciated perhaps most readily in leads II, aVF, and V_1.

2. What does the variation in P-wave configuration and the variation in P-R interval indicate?

ANSWER: The change in configuration of the P wave indicates a variation or a wandering of the location of the atrial pacemaker. If one considers the P-R interval to be a crude caliper representing distance from the origin of the atrial beat to the point of activation of the interventricular septum, the change in P-R interval indicates a change in distance between the atrial pacemaker site and the final common path through the A-V junction, the bundle of His, and the bundle branches. Simplistically one can say that, if the P-R interval is constant and the P-wave configuration varies, the migration or wandering of the atrial pacemaker is along the perimeter of a circle whose radius from the A-V node remains constant. If, on the other hand, the P-R interval varies and the P wave changes very little in configuration, it is most likely that the rate of conduction varies from atrium to ventricle.

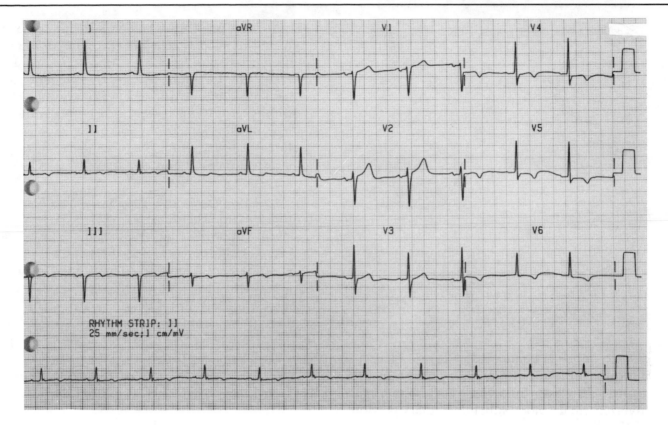

EKG 27

Let us consider the T waves in this record. The record shows no evidence of intraventricular conduction delay and minimal evidence of prolongation of the action potential.

1. How can we make that statement?

ANSWER: As noted on page 55, the *representative* action potential can be calculated by subtracting the QRS duration from the QT interval. In this instance, both the QT interval (.360 sec) and the QRS duration (.08 sec) are within normal limits at a rate of 64 beats per minute. The representative duration of the action potential can be calculated to be .280. Because the QRS configuration and the S-T segments appear to be normal, we can conclude that phase 0, phase 1, and phase 2 of the action potential are normal. Because there is no conduction delay, we can draw the conclusion that the T-wave abnormalities represent derangements of phase 3 of the action potential in some portions of the ventricular myocardium.

2. What are the etiologic possibilities?

ANSWER: One possibility is that each stratum from endocardium to pericardium of the lateral wall of the left ventricle is deficient in repolarizing dipoles, thus generating a deficiency in positive charges facing leads V_4 through V_6 during repolarization (see page 27). If that is the case, the diphasic T wave in lead aVF may be attributed to extension of the lateral myocardial damage into the inferior wall; the involvement there is limited to the

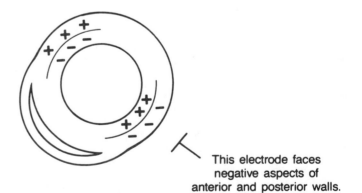

This electrode faces negative aspects of anterior and posterior walls.

Case 27a

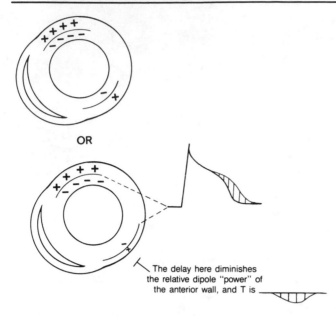

The delay here diminishes the relative dipole "power" of the anterior wall, and T is

Case 27b

deeper, more subendocardial layers. This is indicated by the normal *initial* portion of the diphasic T wave, followed by the abnormal, inverted final (more subendocardial) portion of the T wave.

Another possibility is that ischemic damage to subendocardial cells may produce an island of myocardial cells whose action potentials are *shortened* by ischemia, leading the subendocardial layers to repolarize more rapidly than the healthy, overlying subepicardial myocardium. In that situation, the repolarizing dipoles in the lateral wall would be oriented with their negative poles facing leads V_4 through V_6 (Case 27a).

Because ischemia may instead *prolong* the action potential of damaged cells, the T-wave configuration in leads V_4 through V_6 in this record could represent *delayed* repolarization of all strata of the lateral wall. In that case, the opposite healthy wall repolarizing with its dipoles directed negatively toward leads V_4 through V_6 could at each moment in repolarization direct a more powerful negative charge toward leads V_4 through V_6 than the less developed positive changes directed towards those leads by the lateral myocardium (Case 27b).

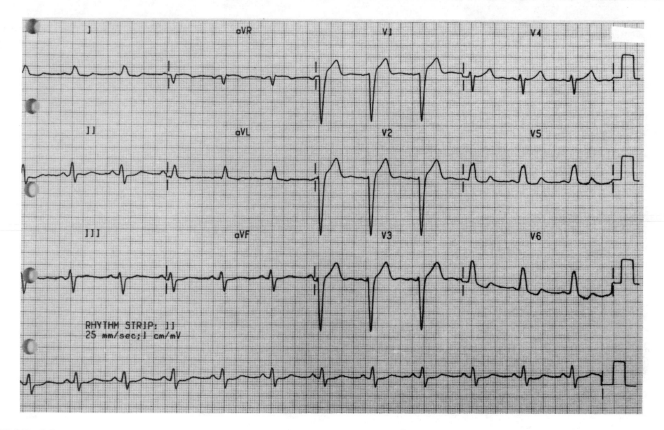

RHYTHM STRIP: II
25 mm/sec; 1 cm/mV

EKG 28

This record indicates an intraventricular conduction delay.

1. Where are the last cells to be depolarized?

ANSWER: Because depolarization advances with positive leading and negative trailing edges, the direction of terminal depolarization is leftward in this record. The last cells to lose their positive surface charges are the source of the final portion of the R wave in the most leftward leads (V_5 and V_6).

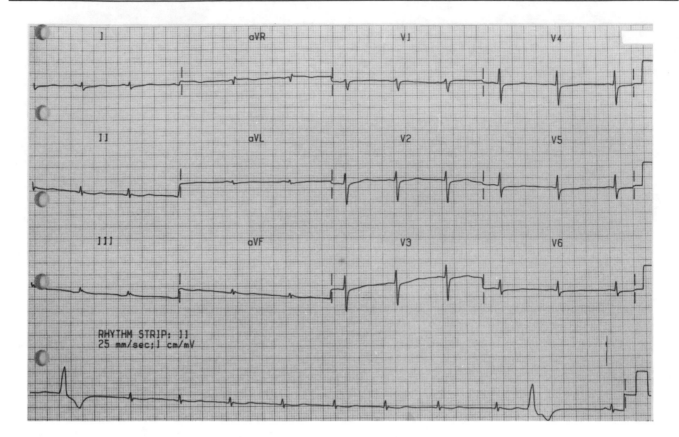

RHYTHM STRIP: II
25 mm/sec; 1 cm/mV

EKG 29

Voltage is low in this record.

1. What are the conventional lower limits of normal in voltage?

ANSWER: Usually, low voltage is recognized when the QRS complexes in the standard leads I, II, and III do not have upward or downward components of at least 5 mm in at least one of the three leads.

In this record, none of the three standard leads I, II, or III has QRS deflection greater than 3 mm.

2. What are the possible causes of this phenomenon in this record?

ANSWER: Low voltage is seen most frequently in the presence of (a) emphysema, in which hyperinflation of the lungs reduces the conductivity of the electric field generated by the heart; (b) massive obesity, in which the excess body mass curtails transport of the electric field to the body surface; or (c) pericardial effusion, in which the low resistance of the effusion induces the electric field to remain concentrated within the confines of the pericardial sac.

Recorded voltage may also be lost or reduced by pleural effusions or myocardial cellular depopulation or infiltration of the myocardium with nonconductive material.

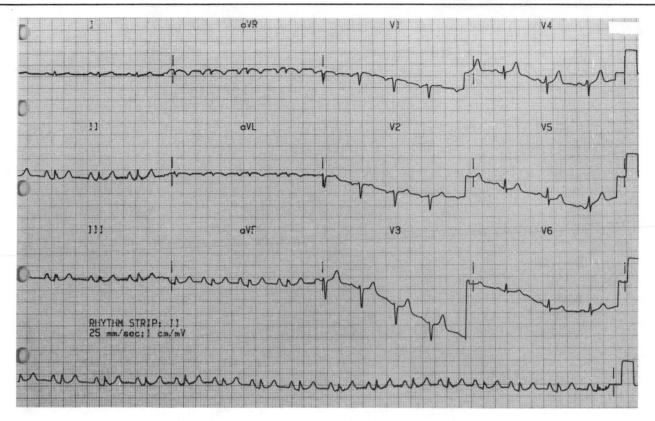

RHYTHM STRIP: II
25 mm/sec; 1 cm/mV

EKG 30

Voltage in this record is also low.

1. Does the record show any clue to the cause of the low voltage?

ANSWER: Prominent P waves with their peaked, almost Christmas-tree profile, are compatible with right atrial enlargement. Therefore, one would consider the possibility of emphysematous pulmonary disease with right heart enlargement to be the most likely explanation for the low voltage.

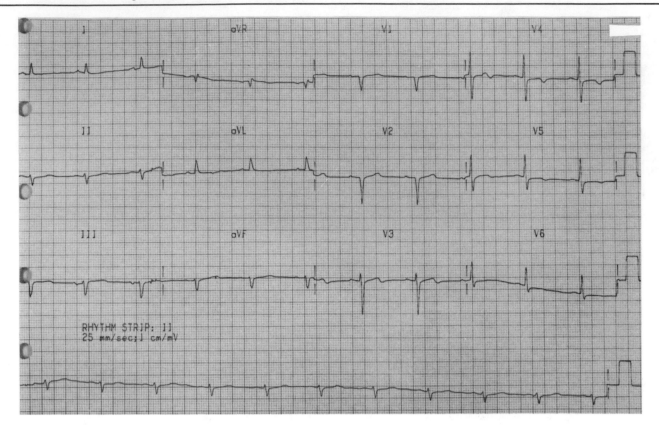

RHYTHM STRIP: II
25 mm/sec; 1 cm/mV

EKG 31

This record has several interesting features. Let us first direct our attention to the T waves in leads V_3 through V_6.

1. What statements would you be willing to make about them?

ANSWER: The symmetrically inverted T wave in lead V_4, and the less inverted T waves in the neighboring leads V_3, V_5, and V_6 suggest that the repolarizing dipole population facing lead V_4 is most severely deficient. That there is a focal concentration of repolarizing abnormality suggests that a discrete area of myocardial damage is located beneath lead V_4.

2. Does S-T,T configuration indicate the age of the process?

ANSWER: Abnormal T waves, like pathologic Q waves, do not indicate the duration of the process without other records for comparison and/or S-T evidence of acute injury. This record gives us no certain indication of the age of the myocardial disease.

3. How do you account for the configuration of leads II, III, aVF, and V_1 through V_3?

ANSWER: The left axis deviation and clockwise rotation are sufficient to be compatible with left anterior hemiblock. The QS configuration in leads V_1 and V_2 may be the result of hemiblock alone or, in addition, may represent anteroseptal myocardial loss at some unknown time.

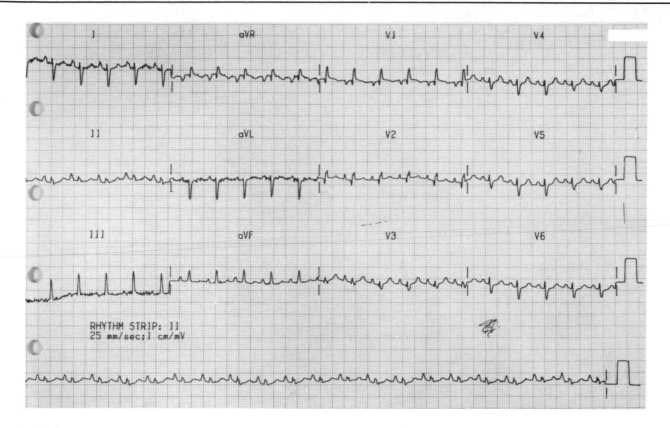

EKG 32

This record has at least three striking features.
1. What are they?
ANSWER: (1) Right axis deviation; (2) tall, peaked, narrow P waves; (3) qR in lead V_1 with rS in lead V_6.

Viewed simply, this record indicates an abnormally large ventricular mass depolarizing toward the right and anteriorly and is a classic presentation of right ventricular hypertrophy. Explanations offered for the three features noted have included marked physical rotation of the heart owing to expansion of the right ventricle against the anterior mediastinum and against the great vessels coursing through the right mediastinum. This theory attributes the large R wave in lead V_1 to rotation so great that the posterior left ventricular wall is directed toward lead V_1. The rS in lead V_6 is similarly related to rotation, so that the cardiac apex faces lead V_6 while the free wall with its terminal depolarization faces posteriorly and rightward.

Some would attribute the Q wave in lead V_1 in this record to septal depolarization in the presence of rotation of the heart to such a degree as to direct the left side of the septum toward lead V_1.

Other explanations have related the late, rightward, and anterior R wave to hypertrophy of the right ventricular free wall and to increased time of conduction over the extended or elongated right ventricular free wall. Some have proposed an increased right ventricular component of the septum, reversing the normal left-to-right septal depolarization to account for the Q wave in leads V_1 and V_2. Right ventricular hypertrophy may be manifested by RSR′ in lead V_1 and S in leads I and V_6 because lengthened conduction up the elongated free wall of the right ventricle may produce prolonged intraventricular conduction as in right bundle branch block.

The tall, narrow P waves in extremity leads are compatible with right atrial dilatation. We should note the negative P waves in lead V_1. Enlargement of the terminal negative portion of the P wave in lead V_1 is an indication of left atrial dilatation. Left atrial enlargement can be expected to *prolong* the P wave, however,

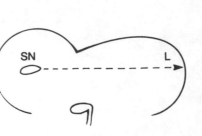
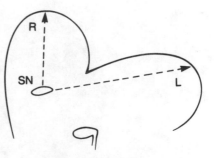
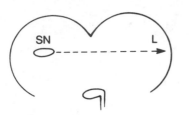

Sinus node—left wall determines normal P-wave duration.	Left atrial enlargement lengthened. SN—left wall axis produces widened P-wave.	Right atrial enlargement may not prolong P-wave

Case 32

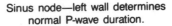

because the transverse diameter from the sinus node to the left wall of the left atrium is elongated. With right atrial enlargement, the overall atrial depolarization time is not prolonged

(Case 32). In this record, the narrow, inverted P wave in lead V_1 can be attributed to clockwise rotation and right atrial enlargement.

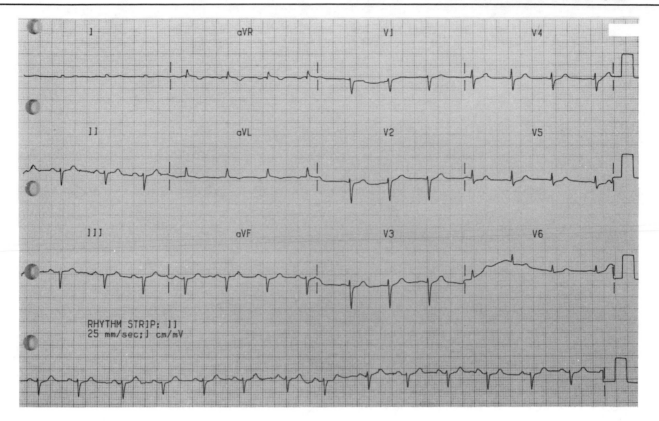

RHYTHM STRIP: II
25 mm/sec; 1 cm/mV

EKG 33

The appearance of rS in leads II, III, and aVF with clockwise rotation in the V leads is indicative of left anterior hemiblock.

1. How would one distinguish this from the electrocardiographic configuration seen after diaphragmatic infarction?

ANSWER: The initial r wave in lead aVF indicates normal depolarization by way of the posterior hemibranch through the intact inferior myocardial wall. After transmural diaphragmatic infarction, this r wave in aVF is replaced by a pathologic Q wave.

2. Suppose the diaphragmatic infarction were small or limited to subendocardium, would the r wave in lead aVF be missing?

ANSWER: A small diaphragmatic myocardial loss might diminish without abolishing the r wave in lead aVF. In such cases, the T wave in aVF may be helpful in distinguishing infarction from anterior hemiblock. The T wave in aVF is upright in hemiblock, because the activation of the diaphragmatic wall occurs without delay; indeed, the inferior wall repolarizes before the anterior and lateral regions, generating an upright T wave in lead aVF. Depletion of repolarizing dipoles in the infarcted diaphragmatic wall, except in very small lesions, generates an inverted T wave.

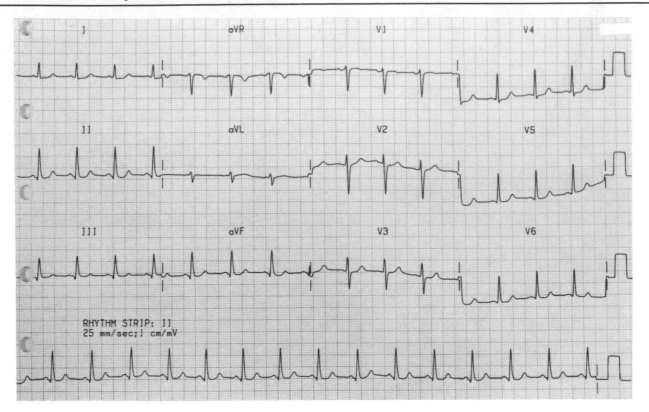

EKG 34

In this record, the S-T segment is depressed in leads I and V$_4$.

1. What is its significance?

ANSWER: Many consider that the normal range of the S-T segment deviation lies between a 2-mm elevation and a .75-mm depression in the V leads. The range is more limited in the extremity leads, where the magnification by proximity is not as powerful. The shape as well as the magnitude of elevation or depression of the S-T segment is an important factor in recognizing normal variants. The concave upward elevated S-T segment with tall T waves (that would "hold water") is much more likely to be a normal variant than is a convex upward elevation.

2. What is the mechanism of the normal concave upward S-T deviation?

ANSWER: Two possibilities have been considered:

(1) A slight variation exists in resting potential among normal myocardial cells. If the heterogeneity is scattered at random through the ventricular myocardium, no net difference develops between regions of the ventricles; thus, no diastolic dipole between cell masses exists. If, however, one region is predominantly different from another (i.e., 86 mV in one area and 94 mV in another), the resultant diastolic dipole would cause the baseline to deviate as in the presence of myocardial injury, and an illusion of S-T deviation would result.

(2) There is regional variation in configuration of phase 2 of the action potential, with repolarization during phase 2 occurring earlier in some areas than in others. Here, the S-T segment would deviate in response to the inequality of simultaneous surface charges during phase 2.

The ST deviations seen in this record may be variants of normal. The record should be repeated if the clinical situation suggests an active process.

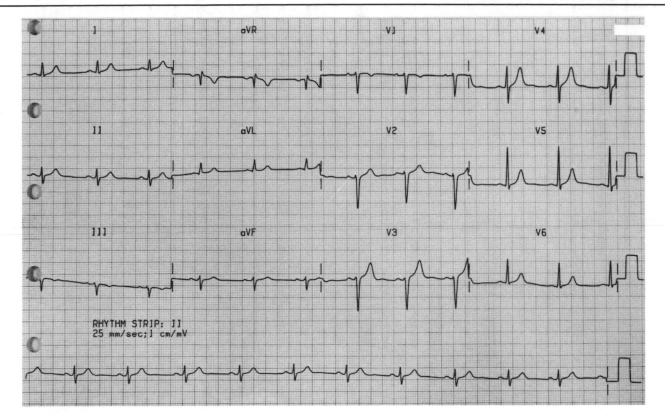

EKG 35

Tall T waves can be seen in this otherwise normal record.

1. What possible mechanisms can produce such peaked, large T waves?

ANSWER: The repolarization wave is the product of the repolarization of the myriad of ventricular cells and is derived from phase 3 of their action potentials. The more steep the slope of phase 3, the greater is the instantaneous difference in charge between cells during the sequential process of repolarization. As discussed on page 26, in a two-cell sample representing an early and a late cell to repolarize in the normal myocardium, the T-wave configuration can be derived readily from the charge difference between the two cells. The normal variation in steepness for phase 3 is considerable with a resulting variation in the height of the normal T wave.

A dramatic, pathologically tall T wave is seen in hyperkalemia, in which phase 3 is very steep, resulting in mountain-peak T waves. Because hyperkalemia is global in its myocardial effects, all leads share the T-wave alteration except aVR in which the T wave becomes abnormally deep. (Lead aVR may be unique in its endocardial vantage point as contrasted with the 11 other leads; thus, normally it registers a negative T wave as repolarization advances from apical epicardium toward endocardium and base). With hyperkalemic repolarization, the steep phase 3s produce a deep T wave in this lead. Tall T waves may be seen in those leads overlying the opposite wall in the presence of focal myocardial damage. Thus, the deeply inverted T wave in lead V_6 in lateral myocardial damage may be associated with a tall peaked T wave in lead V_1. The focal nature of this T wave distinguishes it from hyperkalemia. The tall T wave seen in normal individuals with S-T elevations (as seen in this record) are recognized by the S-T company they keep.

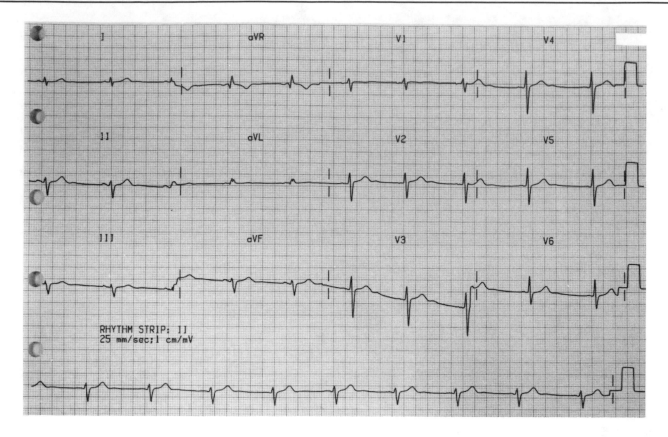

RHYTHM STRIP: II
25 mm/sec; 1 cm/mV

EKG 36

This record presents two diagnostic features produced by left anterior hemiblock.

1. What are they?

ANSWER: Left-axis deviation and clockwise rotation (poor progression of R waves in the precordial leads). After loss of anteriorly and superiorly directed hemibranches, depolarization of the left ventricle is introduced by way of the posterior hemibranch. As described on page 41, invasion of the anterior and lateral walls advances in an apex-to-base and circumferential fashion.

2. The QRS duration here is .10 sec. Would the diagnosis of anterior hemiblock be appropriate if the QRS duration had been normal?

ANSWER: Yes. Many times the QRS duration in hemiblock may be .08 or .09 sec, because this may represent a prolongation of that patient's previous intraventricular conduction time.

3. What is the minimal left-axis deviation seen in the presence of left anterior hemiblock?

ANSWER: Unless the axis is more negative than

—30°, one cannot be confident of left anterior hemiblock.

4. What degree of clockwise rotation is necessary for the diagnosis of left anterior hemiblock?

ANSWER: Usually, one cannot recognize left anterior hemiblock as a solitary abnormality unless there are rS configurations in leads V_2 through V_4 and often in leads V_5 and V_6. As seen on page 42 leads V_1 and V_2 may demonstrate QS or rS complexes.

5. When left anterior hemiblock is combined with incomplete or complete right bundle branch block, what happens to the clockwise rotation?

ANSWER: The appearance of R-S-R' in lead V_1 and often in leads V_2 and V_3 obscures the "poor R-wave progression," but leads V_4 through V_6 continue to reveal qrS or rS. The clue to the combined lesion is the left axis deviation with rS in II and aVF and rS or QS in III in the presence of precordial manifestations of right bundle branch block or incomplete right bundle branch block.

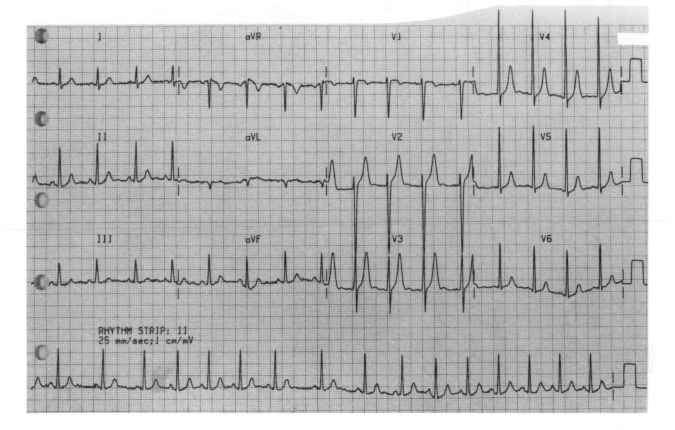

RHYTHM STRIP: II
25 mm/sec;1 cm/mV

EKG 37

Voltage in this record is impressive. Using the familiar formula of S-wave depth (in mm) in lead V_1 plus R-wave height in lead V_5 or V_6, the total is greater than 35 mm.

1. What are the possible diagnoses?

ANSWER: This time-honored formula has been useful in recognizing left ventricular hypertrophy in adult patients of "normal" body build. In young individuals, whose tissues appear to be better conductors than those of adults, the "normal" precordial voltage seen may be greater. Children and adolescents with no sign of cardiac abnormality may generate a voltage of 40 to 45 mm (V_1 S + V_5 or V_6 R = 40 to 45 mm). Occasionally, this juvenile voltage may persist until the person is 20 years old or more. The absence of QRS widening and of S-T,T abnormality is a helpful sign in recognizing this normal variant. A look at the patient can be most helpful, because a thin body build is a potent magnifier of voltage. Indeed, this magnification can occur in older thin individuals as well as in children.

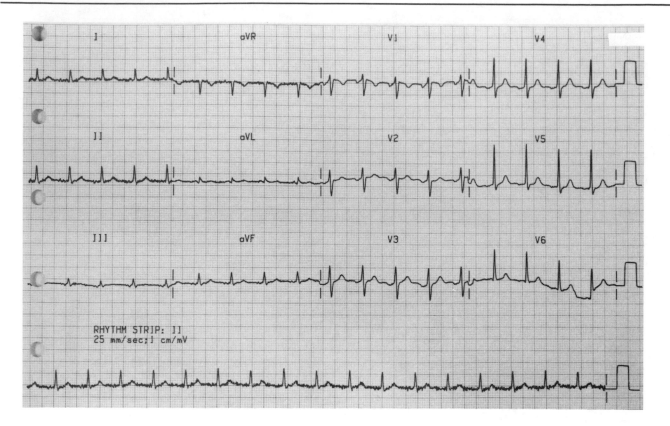

RHYTHM STRIP: II
25 mm/sec;1 cm/mV

EKG 38

Note the P waves and P-R interval. The P waves in leads II, III, and aVF are small and inverted, and in lead aVR they are upright. In the V leads they are inverted.

1. Where is the atrial pacemaker?

ANSWER: Because depolarization advances with a positive leading, and a negative trailing, component, atrial depolarization is advancing here from a caudal and anterior origin. The site must be near the base of the atria near the A-V groove.

2. Does the P-R interval help to identify the pacemaker site?

ANSWER: Yes. Because the P-R interval represents the time course of depolarization from onset of atrial to onset of intraventricular septal activation, it can serve somewhat as a caliper. All atrial pacemaker sites equidistant from the A-V node can be expected to have the same P-R interval, whereas those closer to the A-V node are associated with a shorter P-R interval. Because the P-R interval here (.10 to .11 sec) is less than normal, the site lies closer than normal to the A-V node. Yet, the P-R interval is not sufficiently short to indicate that its position is within the A-V node. Junctional (A-V nodal) rhythm would not be expected to produce a P-R interval greater than .08 to .09 sec; indeed, P-R interval is often lost, with P buried in QRS, or negative, with P following QRS (see page 49). One should be cautious, however. Whenever the P-R interval is short, it is necessary to look for and exclude evidence of an accessory A-V pathway by carefully studying the QRS for delta waves. If the P-R interval is short and the P wave appears normal (indicating a normal pacemaker location), one can recognize accelerated conduction through or around the A-V junction. In the presence of an ectopic atrial pacemaker, however, accelerated A-V conduction can be recognized with certainty only by electrophysiologic studies (see page 49).

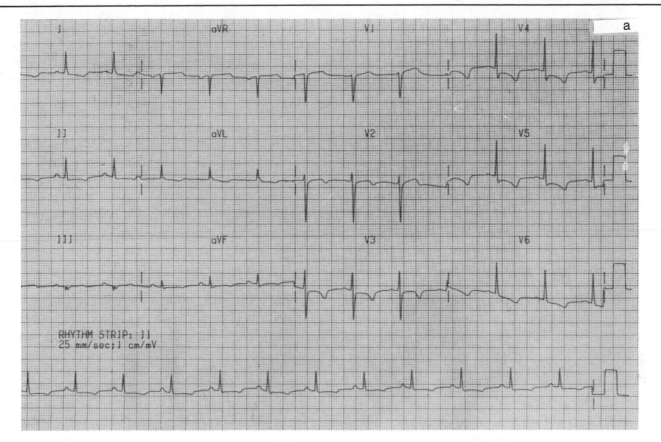

RHYTHM STRIP: II
25 mm/sec; 1 cm/mV

EKG 39

This is a commonly occurring record. One might be content to classify the S-T,T configuration as a nonspecific one.

1. Is this all that one might conclude?

ANSWER: No, it is clinically useful to consider the possibilities that are suggested by this frequently occurring type of tracing. The fundamental message of the record is that repolarization occurs in an abnormal fashion. Those areas of ventricular myocardium in which repolarizing dipoles normally generate positive charges facing diaphragmatic anterior and lateral electrodes are disordered. Are these areas abnormal in their sequence of generation of dipoles because they are the victims of an abnormality in intraventricular conduction? As we have seen in bundle branch block, leads recorded over the delayed areas present inverted T waves because those areas are "handicapped" in the "race to repolarize" by their tardiness in activation. This record gives no indication of intraventricular conduction de-

lay. Does QT evidence of action potential prolongation exist? A localized prolongation of action potential would delay phase 3 repolarization in the affected area and again cause that region to lose the race to repolarize. This record does not reveal QT interval prolongation. (A QT of .40 sec at a rate of 72 to 73 beats per minute is at the extreme upper limit of normal.) We can then consider other possibilities. If the interior, anterior, and lateral myocardium were damaged so as to reduce the population of sarcolemmal dipoles, those areas would lose the repolarization race. Let us push this possibility further: If the stratum of depleted inferior and anterolateral myocardium was subepicardial, the early portion of the T wave would be inverted in leads facing this area; if instead, the depopulation affected only the subendocardial layer, the terminal portion of the repolarization race would be lost by this area, and terminal T-wave invasion would be seen in the overlying leads. If the cell loss were transmural in an area, the affected region would lose the race throughout repolarization and the T waves in overlying leads would be totally inverted.

2. Would the depth of T-wave inversion have a quantitative significance?

ANSWER: Yes. The greater the loss of sarcolemmal repolarization, the greater the T-wave inversion.

3. We are considering the possibility that this record represents sarcolemmal loss in the inferior, anterior, and lateral walls. Yet there is no QRS indication of gross loss of myocardium by infarction. Isn't this contradictory?

ANSWER: No. We are not suggesting a region of cell loss of gross proportions but, instead, a sufficiently diffuse micro-loss of sarcolemma to be recognizable in the "spread-out process of repolarization." This loss of sarcolemmal activity would not be sufficient to be recognizable in the "compact" sequence of depolarization. A nonphysiologic analogy might be relevant here: If a herd of horses stampeded by your grandstand, you probably would not be able to detect a few missing animals; if, however, the herd were strung out and ran by you more slowly, the absence of some animals would be noticed.

Often, records such as this represent subendocardial infarction. In this situation, the gross area of myocardial loss may be limited to the subendocardial self-cancelling stratum discussed earlier, and no pathologic Q wave would appear. The overlying, less dense myocardial damage might be reflected in the totally inverted T wave.

4. Often, records like this are found in a series of tracings with rapidly changing T-wave abnormalities. Is there an explanation for the T-wave configurations in those situations?

ANSWER: Because an actively damaged cell may leak its K^+ more rapidly and phase 3 may be inscribed earlier and more steeply, the sequences of repolarization may be impressively altered. If subendocardial and mid-wall ischemic damage causes those layers to repolarize more rapidly than the more normal superficial strata, leads over this area will be faced with negative aspects of the repolarizing dipoles generated in the affected wall as well as the negative poles of the normal opposite wall (Case 39). Thus, these leads will record inverted T waves. If the process fluctuates in intensity, the T wave fluctuates in form and depth.

5. If such an acute process were transmural, what would the overlying leads register?

ANSWER: During the acute period, the early repolarization of the affected wall could generate pathologically tall T waves in overlying leads. As the process evolved with more loss of sarcolemmal activity as a result of damage, the T-wave would become inverted.

6. Does the S-T depression in leads V_5 and V_6 have significance?

ANSWER: It is a signal that sarcolemmal insult has probably been sufficient to reduce the resting potential (see page 28). Because cell damage to the point of reduction of resting potential usually does not persist, the cell either dies or is rescued from the intense damage by physiologic or therapeutic means. Such S-T deviations in the presence of these T-wave abnormalities justify further records if there is clinical suspicion of an active process.

This patient's EKG was recorded following 7 days of unstable angina pectoris. On the day of this recording, cardiac catheterization re-

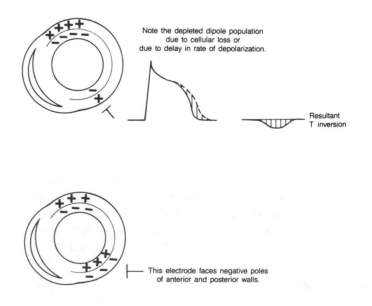

Note the depleted dipole population due to cellular loss or due to delay in rate of depolarization.

Resultant T inversion

This electrode faces negative poles of anterior and posterior walls.

Case 39

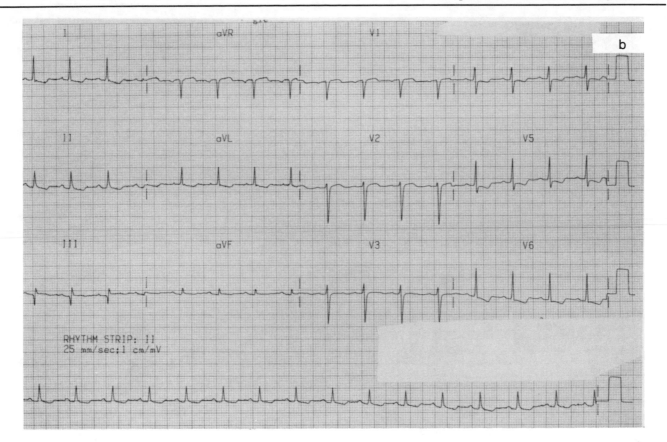

vealed 100% occlusion of the left anterior descending, 70% obstruction of the left main, 60% obstruction of the circumflex, and 90% obstruction of the right coronary artery. The patient was subsequently subjected to coronary bypass surgery. The postoperative electrocardiogram (39b) showed improvement in the S-T,T configuration.

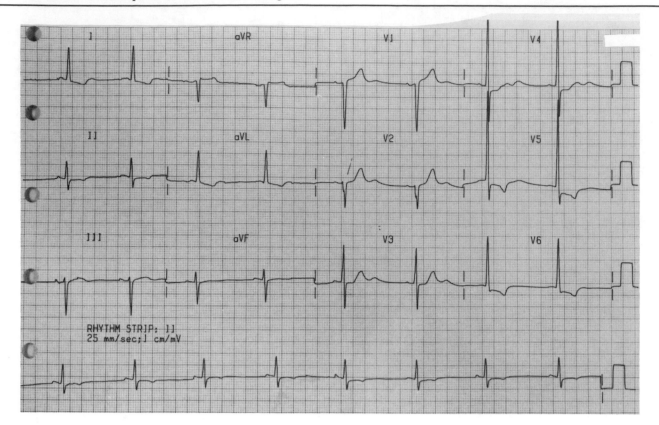

EKG 40

Left ventricular hypertrophy has produced considerable increase in QRS voltage in this record. In addition, the S-T,T configurations are abnormal.

1. Are they related to the ventricular enlargement?

ANSWER: The downsloping S-T and low upright terminal T waves in leads I and aVL are typical of the configurations seen in the presence of left ventricular hypertrophy. As noted on page 65, this S-T,T configuration is the most sensitive EKG indicator of left ventricular hypertrophy, but is nonspecific because it may be produced by interventricular block, digitalis, sympathomimetic stimulation, and hypercalcemia (page 65). The S-T,T in leads V_5 and V_6 is also nonspecific. It may represent deformity of the action potential produced by enlargement of myocardial cells. On the basis of this single record, however, one could not exclude the possibility that the full-length S-T depressions are the result of ischemic loss of resting potential of anterolateral subendocardial myocardium or of posteromedial trans-

mural myocardium (page 28). Nor could one exclude the possibility that the sharply inverted T waves in these leads reflect ischemic alteration in phase 3 (pages 27 and 28). Clinical information and serial records would be necessary to recognize an active ischemic process in the presence of left ventricular hypertrophy. Often, serial records in the presence of left ventricular hypertrophy show a constant, unchanging S-T,T configuration as seen in leads V_5 and V_6.

One may speculate further on the mecha-

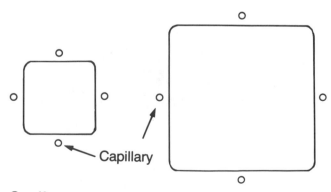

Case 40

nisms involved: (a) Enlargement of left ventricular myocardial cells might alter phases 2 and 3 of the action potential by unknown means. (b) The extended distance between pericellular capillaries and the center of hypertrophied cells might, without coronary artery disease, generate cellular ischemia with resultant phase 2 and 3 modification (Case 40). (c) Ventricular hypertrophy is often complicated by coronary disease. (d) In many instances, left ventricular hypertrophy is associated with prolongation of intraventricular conduction significant enough to alter S-T,T in the same fashion as seen in left bundle branch block. The present record does not indicate such a delay.

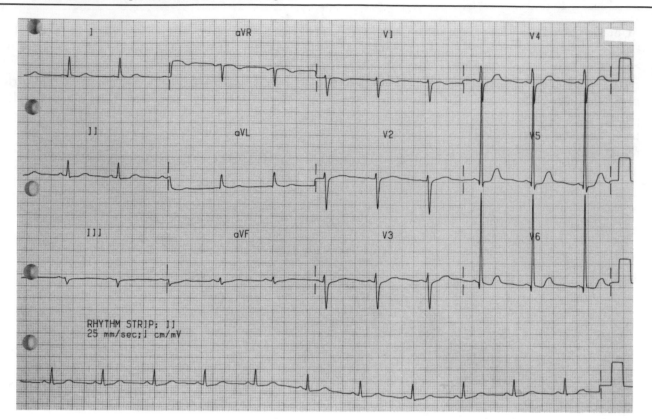

RHYTHM STRIP: II
25 mm/sec;1 cm/mV

EKG 41

This might be considered a standard presentation of left ventricular hypertrophy with (a) increased voltage, (b) prolonged intraventricular conduction, (c) downsloping S-T,T in left-sided leads, and (d) diphasic T waves with upright terminal configuration in left-sided leads.

1. If 100 hearts had left ventricular hypertrophy at autopsy, how many would have shown all 4 electrocardiographic features?

ANSWER: Less than 50—probably 20 or so. Approximately 40 would present only the nonspecific S-T,T configuration discussed under "left ventricular strain" (page 65). Fre-

quently, left ventricular hypertrophy is manifested by an increase in voltage and by the S-T,T configuration as seen here, without prolongation of QRS duration. If we recall that intraventricular conduction time normally begins with septal depolarization and terminates with depolarization of the base of the free wall of the left ventricle, left ventricular hypertrophy that has not produced lengthening of the distance between the terminal Purkinje twigs and the base of the heart may not prolong intraventricular conduction despite thickening of the ventricular wall.

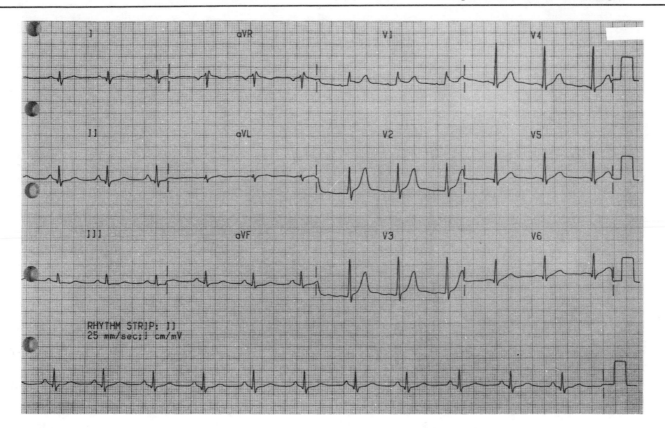

RHYTHM STRIP: II
25 mm/sec;1 cm/mV

EKG 42

The notched R in lead V_1, Rs in leads V_2 and V_3, qRs in leads V_4 through V_6, the qRs in leads I and II, and the large, tall T waves in leads V_1 through V_3 are some of the striking features of this record.

1. What are the basic messages of this record?

ANSWER: We could start as follows: excessive positive depolarization forces are directed anteriorly. Note that they are not limited to the *right anterior* quadrant as seen in easy-to-recognize right ventricular hypertrophy with a tall R wave in lead V_1 and rS in leads V_2 and V_3. The record suggests either an increase in dipole population of the anterior wall of the heart or a loss of some posterior cell population. The tall T waves in leads V_2 and V_3 support the possibility of posterior myocardial loss and suggest that the examination of posterior leads would reveal deeply inverted ischemic-type T waves. Thus, the record brings to mind the possibility of posterior infarction. Before we become too confident, however, we must consider other features of this record. Duration of the QRS (ventricular conduction time) is prolonged and S waves occur in leads I, aVL, aVF, and V_2 through V_6 and rSr' in aVR. The final depolarization process, therefore, is directed posteriorly and to the right. Is this incomplete right bundle branch block? If so, the QRS in lead V_1 demands study. Why is there a notched R wave and not RSR' as would be expected in right bundle branch block? If, in fact, there has been posterior myocardial loss, the disappearance of the S wave in the RSR' in V_1 would be accounted for. We have often seen this configuration following posterior infarction complicated by right bundle branch block. We have not often seen this record with its Rs segment in leads V_2 and V_3 as a result of right ventricular hypertrophy.

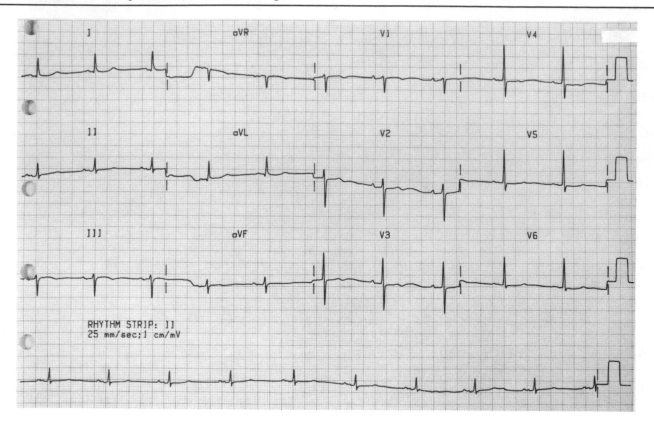

EKG 43

Notched wide P waves (.12 sec) indicate left atrial enlargement.

1. What added information is gained from the abnormal S-T,T configuration?

ANSWER: Normally, T waves are upright in leads facing the apex and the anterior and left lateral walls of the heart. The T waves seen here are nonspecific, but they suggest ventricular myocardial abnormality that is not focal or regional. It is important to recognize that they do not include S-T,T characteristics produced by deformity of the second portions of phase 2 and phase 3 following digitalis action, nor do they reveal the prolongation of phase 2 with S-T prolongation and sagging generated by quinidine and its relatives or by hypokalemia. It is the combination of P and S-T,T abnormalities here that tells the story of left ventricular damage even though it does not, of course, reveal the type of that damage.

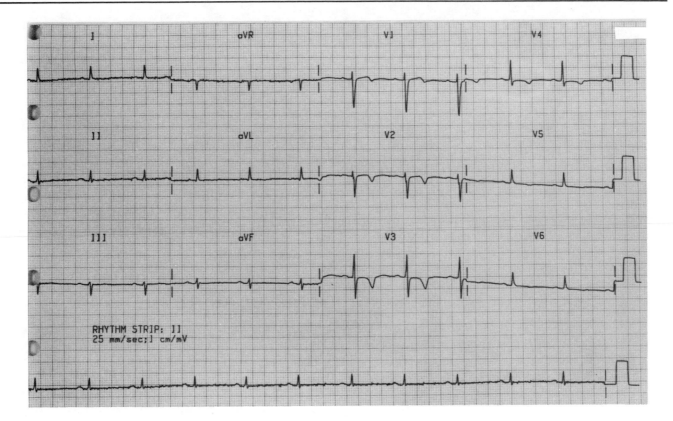

EKG 44

The point of presenting this record is to consider the T configuration in the V leads. They are symmetrical and most deeply inverted in lead V_3 with inversion decreasing to the right and left of that lead.

1. Could this be a normal variant?

ANSWER: By no means. It is important to visualize the ventricles as a horseshoe-shaped structure divided longitudinally by the interventricular septum. Lead V_1 lies over the right corner of the base of the horseshoe. As repolarization advances from the apical-septal area, it is as though the positive charge appears first at the apex of the horseshoe and advances up its arms and septum toward the base (Case 44). Normally, the horseshoe may be positioned so that lead V_1 lies in the negative field generated by repolarization. Leads V_2, V_3, and V_4 however, are progressively nearer the apex of the horseshoe and, therefore, are in a progressively more positive field during repolarization. T waves in normal individuals, therefore, may be inverted in lead V_1, sometimes in lead V_2, and rarely in lead V_3; but in

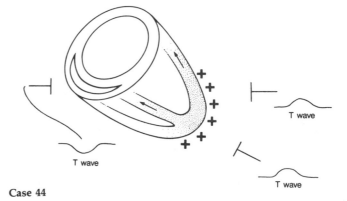

Case 44

those normal cases, the T waves are less negative in lead V_2 than they are in lead V_1, and less in V_3 than in V_2. Thus, T waves normally progress toward upright in leads V_1 through V_3 and are upright in leads V_4 through V_6. Often, the tallest T wave is in lead V_4 in normal persons, because the electrode lies at the apex of the horseshoe. When T waves grow deeper from leads V_1 to V_2 to V_3, as in this record, some process has depleted repolarization dipole population in the anteroseptal, anterior region. Most often, this record is seen in ischemic myocardial disease.

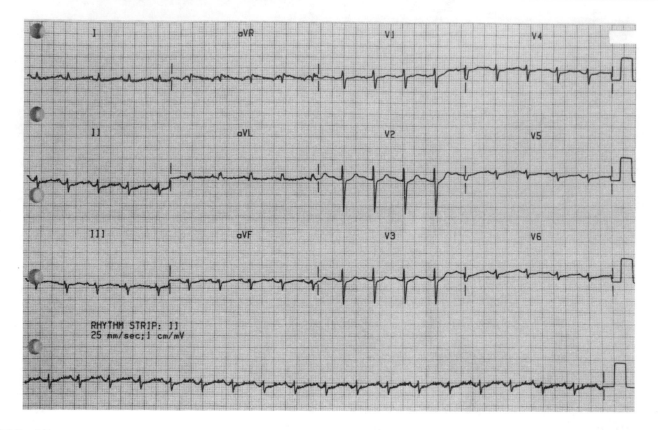

RHYTHM STRIP: II
25 mm/sec; 1 cm/mV

EKG 45

This record shows low voltage, left-axis deviation, clockwise rotation, and slight S-T depression in leads V_2 through V_6.

1. How far do you go with interpretations of this record?

ANSWER: We have considered the causes of loss of voltage. This patient might be obese, emphysematous, or afflicted with pericardial effusion or a myocardial infiltrative or depopulating disease. The left-axis deviation with clockwise rotation is suggestive of left anterior hemiblock. The S-T depressions are marginal (reasonable normal range is 0 to .75 mm in V leads). One would wisely report these features and obtain other information if other processes were suspected. Careful observation of S-T,T changes in future records is important.

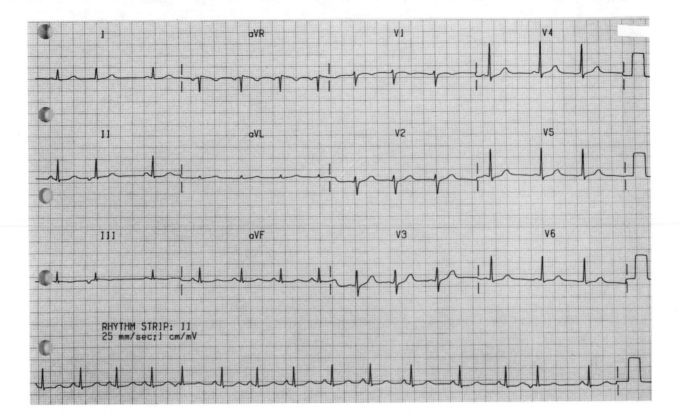

RHYTHM STRIP: II
25 mm/sec;1 cm/mV

EKG 46

Twice in this record P waves change and P-R interval lengthens slightly.

1. What is this?

ANSWER: Atrial premature contractions occur twice from a single focus. That focus lies in the basal region of the atria and depolarization advances from the caudal toward the cranial region of the atria. The lengthened P-R interval suggests two explanations: the focus is farther from the A-V node than the normal site is (in the S-A node) or the conduction pathway is slower than the normal S-A/A-V nodal paths.

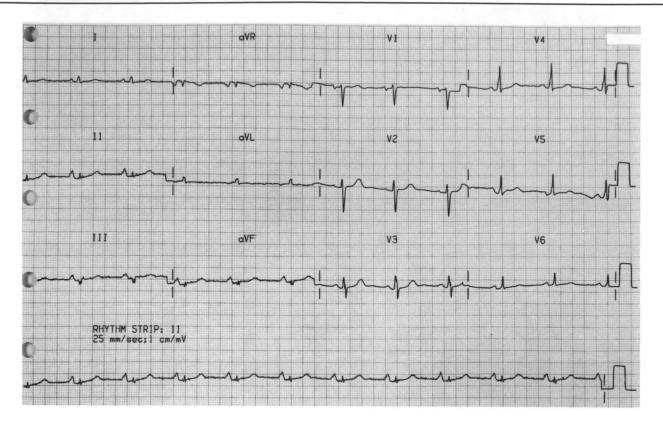

EKG 47

Low voltage and narrow, peaked P waves are a common combination recorded in one section of the hospital.

1. Which would it be?

ANSWER: The pulmonary service. The tall P wave of Christmas tree silhouette and narrow base results from enlargement of the right atrium. Because the duration of the P wave is determined by the conduction time from the S-A node to the most remote portion of the opposite (left) atrium (page 117), enlargement of the proximal atrium does not broaden the P wave unless right atrial dilatation is massive. Loss of voltage completes the combination of abnormalities resulting from obstructive pulmonary disease.

2. There is a small Q wave in lead aVF. Does this indicate diaphragmatic infarction?

ANSWER: Q waves less than .04 sec in duration are not *diagnostic* of myocardial loss. In my experience, the duration of the Q wave has been much more important than its depth in discerning infarction. Admittedly, minor loss of cell population by infarction may occur without pathologic (.04-sec) Q waves; often, in such instances, symmetrically inverted T waves, or reduction in R wave height since earlier records, may be the indicators of cell loss.

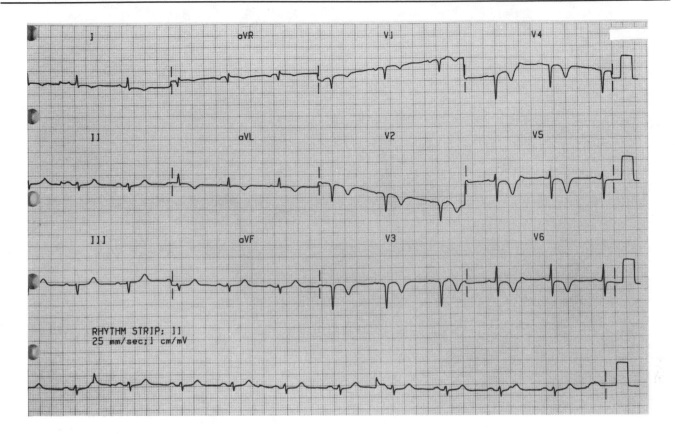

RHYTHM STRIP: 11
25 mm/sec; 1 cm/mV

EKG 48

Loss of normal depolarization positivity (loss of normal R waves) and loss of normal repolarization positivity (loss of upright T waves) have produced a strikingly abnormal record here.

1. What is the problem?

ANSWER: The loss of depolarizing and repolarizing dipoles here indicates loss of sarcolemmal function and implies loss of cells in the regions facing leads V_1 through V_6. Thus, there has been an extensive anteroseptal, anterior, and lateral loss of myocardial cells. We would immediately attribute this to infarction realizing all the while that a bullet wound, a metastasis, an abscess or any other "space - taking process" could be responsible.

2. What is the meaning of the smaller-than-normal R waves in leads V_5 and V_6?

ANSWER: Compared with the myocardium facing leads V_2 through V_4, less depopulation of cells has occurred in this "outer suburb" of the infarction.

3. Does the QS in leads V_1 through V_4 mean all cells are gone in that area?

ANSWER: No. We have seen active, asymptomatic patients with such records. The appearance of the QS *does* mean cell loss has been severe enough to cause the dipole population (and, therefore, the cell population) facing anteriorly to be less numerous than that facing posteriorly. But the QS does not mean total loss of cells.

The T waves are deeply inverted in a wider area of V leads than are the QS waves.

4. How can this be?

ANSWER: Once again, T-wave sensitivity to cell damage or loss has been shown to be greater than QRS sensitivity (page 28). This marginal area of the infarction has been damaged sufficiently to yield T-wave inversion, but only to reduce the amplitude of the R wave.

Left axis deviation with clockwise rotation suggests left anterior hemiblock.

5. Is that likely here?

ANSWER: Yes. The infarct lies across the pathways of the anterior hemibranch.

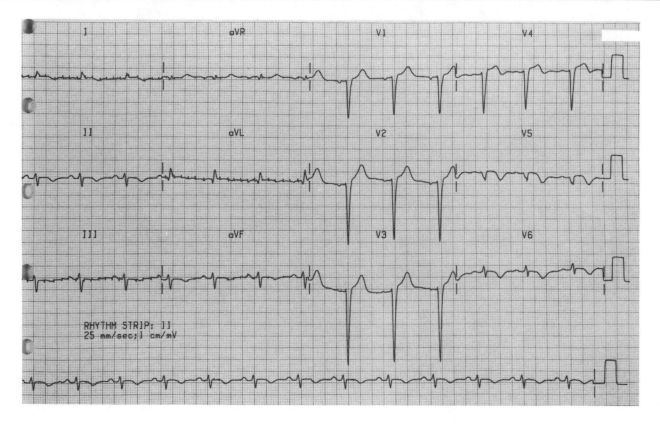

RHYTHM STRIP: II
25 mm/sec; 1 cm/mV

EKG 49

This record resembles the previous record but there are rS in leads V_1 through V_4, tiny rS in lead V_5 and rs in lead V_6, and T waves are inverted in leads V_5 and V_6 and in leads I, II, III, and aVF.

1. How does the lesion here differ from the previous record?

ANSWER: The persistence of small R waves in leads V_1 through V_5 implies a greater population of surviving cells in the matrix of this infarct than in the previous record. The center of greatest destruction lies under lead V_5, whereas the ring of less massive ischemic damage extends into the inferior wall.

Again, there is left axis deviation with clock-wise rotation compatible with left anterior hemiblock. Voltage is at the lower limit of normal in extremity leads, probably, in this case, a result of loss of myocardium. The slight S-T elevation in leads I and aVL is noteworthy.

2. What might they represent?

ANSWER: If no previous records exist for comparison, and especially if there is clinical suspicion of recent damage, these minor S-T elevations would justify further electrocardiograms to study the possibility of an active ischemic injury. Indeed, further records and clinical data might confirm that the infarct occurred recently.

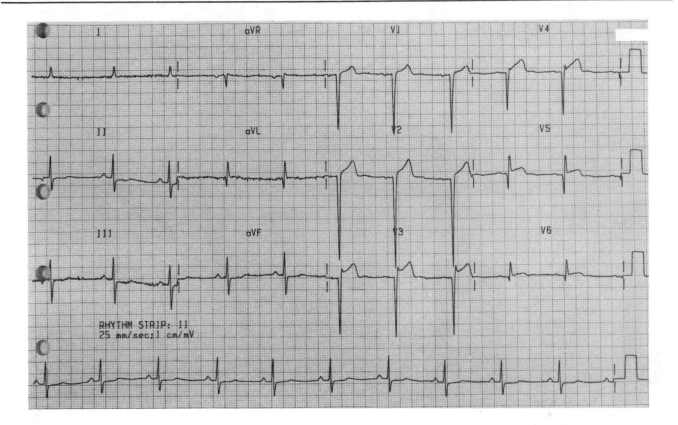

RHYTHM STRIP: II
25 mm/sec; 1 cm/mV

EKG 50

1. Is this anteroseptal anterior infarction active?

ANSWER: Based on this single record, one would conclude from the S-T deviations that there is a population of myocardial cells with subnormal resting potential or abnormal phase 2 of action potential (pages 28 and 102). Three important possibilities are presented: (1) This is an acute infarction with a population of severely injured cells in the necrotic lesion. (2) This is an old infarction, now afflicted by a fresh episode of ischemic injury. (3) This is an old infarction which is aneurysmal: the stretched sarcolemma of the thinned wall producing chronically leaky cells with lower than normal resting potential.

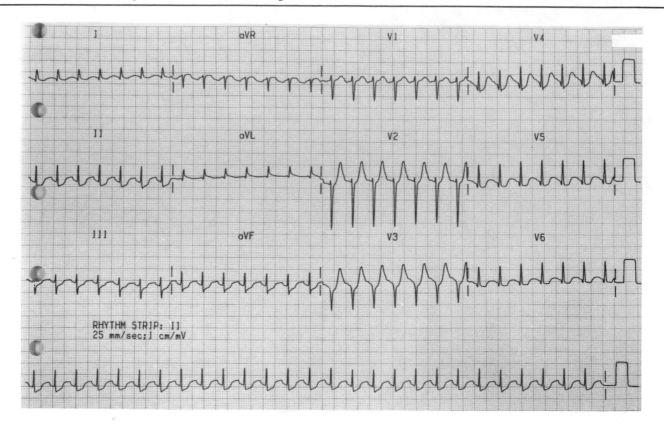

RHYTHM STRIP: II
25 mm/sec;1 cm/mV

EKG 51

This is another anterior infarction with a QS segment in lead V_3. The nearly horizontal S-T deviation in leads II, III, aVF, and V_3 through V_5 and the tall T waves in leads V_2 and V_3 require consideration.

1. What do they suggest?
ANSWER: The S-T segments suggest a colony of severely distressed cells with subnormal resting potential (pages 28 to 35) in the subendocardium of the inferior and anterior wall or in the posterior transmural region.

Further records would help analyze the T waves. They may be reciprocal evidence of posterior cell damage or they might represent acute, fresh anteroseptal anterior ischemia (page 126). If succeeding records revealed T-wave inversion in leads V_2 and V_3, one could reasonably conclude the tall T waves were indicators of fresh ischemic damage; if later records showed persistent or increasing T height, a posterior lesion would be expected.

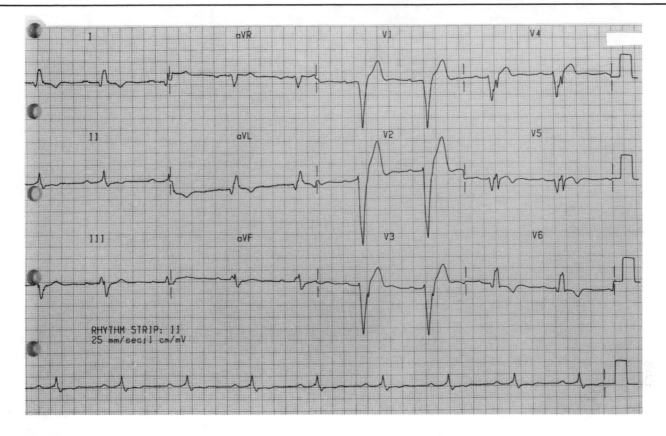

I   aVR   V1   V4

II   aVL   V2   V5

III   aVF   V3   V6

RHYTHM STRIP: II
25 mm/sec; 1 cm/mV

EKG 52

This anterior and lateral infarction is complicated by some process that has lengthened the intraventricular conduction time to .16 to .17 sec.

1. What is the problem?

ANSWER: Peri-infarction conduction delay is recognized by the occurrence of delayed R wave following a pathologic Q wave. As seen here in leads I, aVL, V_5, and V_6, one can read-ily imagine the depolarization process "picking its way" through and around the debris of infarction, with the final depolarizing dipoles facing those leads which overlie the infarction. The configuration in lead V_5 might permit one to visualize the advance of the depolarizing dipoles around and among the strata of living and dead cells in the lesion.

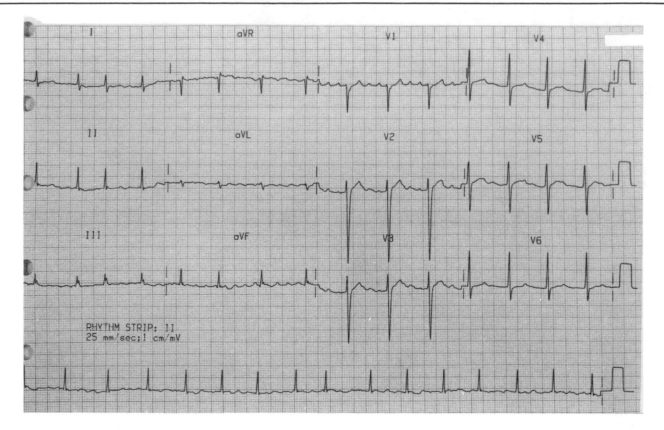

EKG 53

1. Is the atrial rhythm fibrillation, flutter, or tachycardia?

ANSWER: The constant configuration and regularity of the atrial waves excludes fibrillation. The atrial rate of 340 beats per minute falls within the limits generally attributed to flutter (250 to 350 beats per minute). This record illustrates that the electrocardiographic distinction between flutter and tachycardia may be difficult, and indeed, arbitrary. The isoelectric baseline between atrial waves in lead V_1 in this record suggests a diastolic period between atrial depolarizations such as seen in supraventricular tachycardia. A rapidly-firing ectopic focus could generate the record seen here. Flutter, on the other hand, as a circus or re-entry rhythm, should more typically produce a constantly undulating atrial record. The possibility of overlap is readily appreciated. A unifocal tachycardia, generated so rapidly as to release the succeeding depolarization before the previous wave has completed its migration would produce an undulating or "picket-fence" flutter-type record. On the other hand, re-entry or circus pathways that include segments oriented at 90° to the lead might be represented by atrial waves separated by flat isoelectric segments.

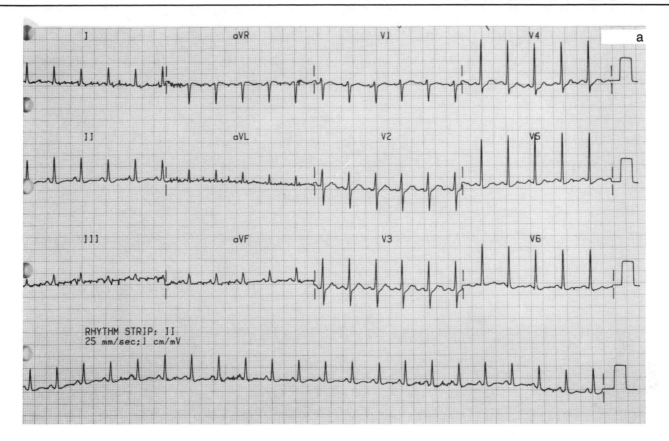

RHYTHM STRIP: II
25 mm/sec; 1 cm/mV

EKG 54

Sinus tachycardia is associated with shortening of the Q-T interval. In this record, at a rate of 132 beats per minute, with the Q-T interval of .200 to .240, the abbreviated Q-T interval is shorter than can be expected on the basis of rate alone.

1. What possibilities could generate this record with a short Q-T interval and J-point depression with S-T depression?

ANSWER: (a) Sympathomimetic effects on the action potential include increased downsloping of phase 2 and shortening of duration, commonly reflected in configurations such as seen here. (b) Hypercalcemia abbreviates phase 2 and remarkably shortens the action potential, producing electrocardiographic abnormalities rather like those from digitalis. In our experience, the brief, downsloping S-T segment in hypercalcemia is more striking than the configuration produced by digitalis. The present record differs from the hypercalcemic record in that the S-T is not sharply downsloping. (c) Whereas digitalis produces a downsloping S-T and shortens the Q-T, in this record the S-T is too brief and S-Ts are not downsloping.

At the time EKG 54a was recorded, the patient was in acute respiratory distress, had pulled out her endotracheal tube, and was receiving atropine by injection and epinephrine by inhalation. Serum calcium concentration was 9.0. She had received no digitalis. When the second electrocardiogram (54b) was recorded on the following day, the crisis had passed, catecholamine administration had ceased, and S-T, T and Q-T abnormalities had disappeared. Thus the abnormalities seen on the first record appear to have been the result of endogenous and exogenous sympathomimetic factors.

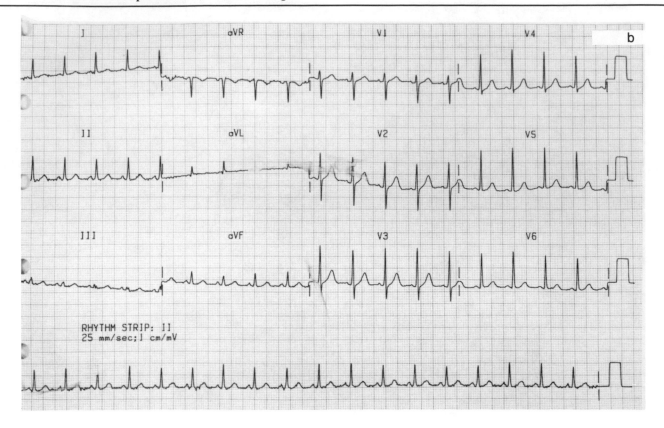

RHYTHM STRIP: II
25 mm/sec; 1 cm/mV

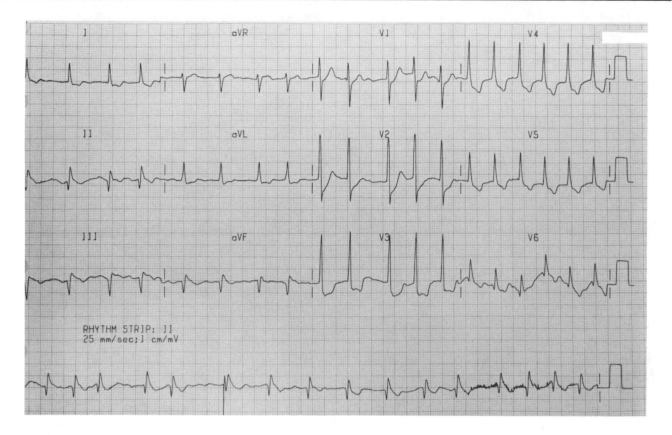

RHYTHM STRIP: II
25 mm/sec; 1 cm/mV

EKG 55

The occurrences of Qr in leads II, III, and aVF and of prominent R waves in leads V_1 through V_3 are indicative of diaphragmatic-posterior myocardial loss. This patient was an elderly woman who had had severe chronic obstructive pulmonary disease and was admitted to the hospital deeply cyanotic with clinical evidence of acute pulmonary insufficiency.

1. To what might one attribute the deep S-T depression in leads V_2 and V_3?

ANSWER: They may represent acute posterior myocardial injury. Without clinical information and additional tracings, we cannot know whether this represents the acute sarcolemmal injury in acute infarction, or whether this is fresh injury in the presence of an old infarction. In this patient with an old posterior infarction, the occurrence of severe generalized hypoxia may have precipitated posterior myocardial injury without new coronary obstructive event.

2. Could the tall R waves in leads V_2 and V_3 be the result of right ventricular enlargement rather than of posterior infarction?

ANSWER: Right ventricular enlargement is most productive of tall R waves in lead V_1 followed by rS in lead V_2, with progressive enlargement of the R waves in leads V_3 through V_6. The reverse is seen here with taller R waves in leads V_2 and V_3. This record, in my opinion, indicates posterior inferior infarction.

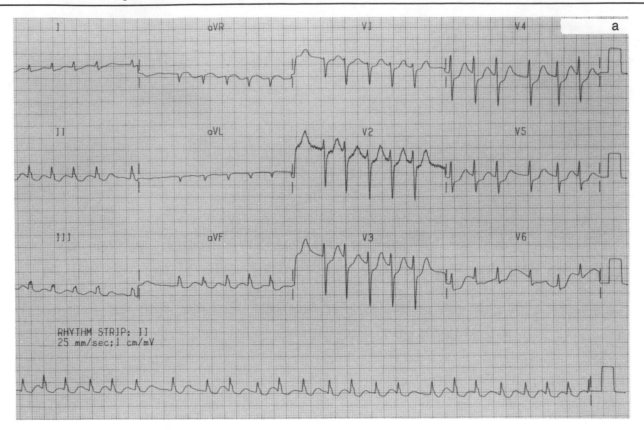

EKG 56

On June 15 this patient was in near-terminal state, in shock and pulmonary edema. PO_2 was 53 mm Hg, pulmonary capillary wedge pressure was 37 mm Hg. Atrial rhythm was fibrillation.

1. What is the meaning of the S-T,T configuration in EKG 56a?

ANSWER: The nearly horizontally depressed S-T segments in leads V_1 through V_6 are compatible with reduction of resting potential in a widespread anterior subendocardial region or in an equally widespread transmural posterior region (see page 35). Resting potential depends on the integrity of the sarcolemma and its Na-K ATPase. In this case, the abnormality can reasonably be attributed to ischemic injury of the sarcolemma. As in many situations, these S-T abnormalities may be the electrocardiographic correlates of regional pallor or cyanosis, acidosis, and hypokinesis.

Horizontal S-T deviations are often seen in such situations and are frequent indicators of myocardial ischemia in the presence of generalized hypoxia or hypoperfusion.

The following day the patient had improved significantly, and shock and pulmonary edema had subsided (EKG 56b).

2. What do the S-T,T changes indicate?

ANSWER: They are compatible with restoration of more nearly normal sarcolemmal function. One can reasonably conclude that the myocardial cyanosis or pallor has subsided.

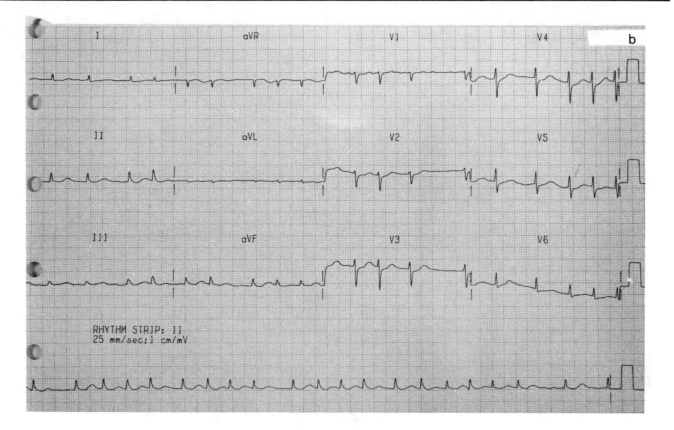

RHYTHM STRIP: II
25 mm/sec;1 cm/mV

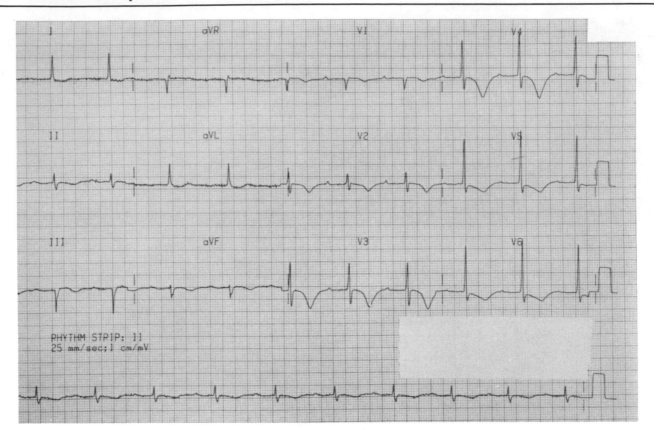

EKG 57

Ischemic damage has been found to shorten or to lengthen the action potential in laboratory studies, and many clinical records appear to confirm this belief.

In this record, inverted T waves and markedly prolonged Q-T interval (.52 sec, at a rate of 63 beats per minute) occur without prolongation of QRS complex. The prolongation is in the J-T interval.

1. What is the J-T interval? What is its duration here?

ANSWER: The J-T interval is the duration of the action potential of a representative myocardial cell (page 55). Here, its duration is significantly prolonged (.44 sec).

2. What possible causes come to mind?

ANSWER: (a) Hypokalemia might produce such a record, but clinical data do not indicate a potassium deficit. Serum potassium level on the day of this record was 3.8 to 4.2 mEq/L.

(b) Quinidine, procainamide, and disopyramide prolong the Q-T and J-T intervals, but do not cause the deeply inverted, symmetrical T waves seen here.

(c) Central nervous system (CNS) disorders with associated autonomic dysfunction may produce this type of record (page 66). There was no sign of CNS disorder in this case.

(d) This record occurred in the clinical setting of acute myocardial ischemia and appears to illustrate ischemic prolongation of the action potential.

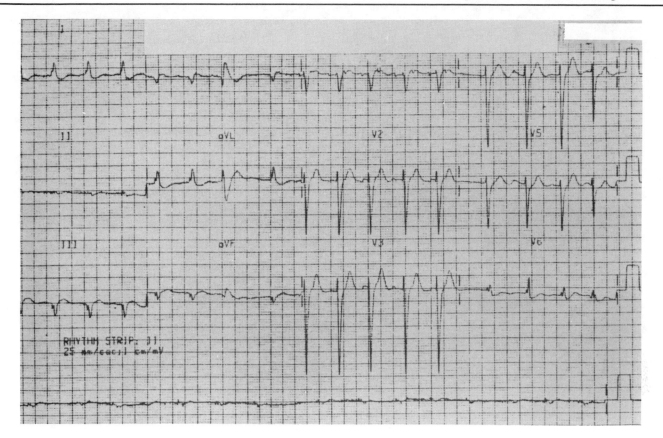

EKG 58

The atrial rate is 240 beats per minute with regular rhythm and 2:1 A-V block. The baseline between atrial waves is flat and the atrial waves are negative in the only leads in which they are well seen (V_1, V_2, and V_3).

1. What mechanisms might produce this atrial arrhythmia?

ANSWER: This record illustrates the difficulty of imposing rigid definitions on some arrhythmic records and the importance of visualizing fundamental mechanisms. If this record were considered to represent atrial flutter with a rate of 240 beats per minute, the prolonged apparent isoelectric period between atrial waves would require a circus pathway lying in two planes intersecting at 90°. Probably the minor portion of the reentry loop would course in the plane registered by lead V_1. The major portion of the loop would course in the plane at 90° to the axis and therefore be unregistered by lead V_1.

A micro-circus pathway located in the atria with centrifugal waves extending anteriorly and posteriorly might equally well produce the configuration seen in lead V_1.

The final possibility is that this record represents an ectopic automatic focus in the atria. Without intracardiac recordings, the identification of the process remains debatable.

In many atrial arrhythmias, the atrial waves are seen best in inferior leads aVF and III as well as in V_1 because reentry loops are frequently directed in an oblique plane from the right inferior to the left superior portion of the atria.

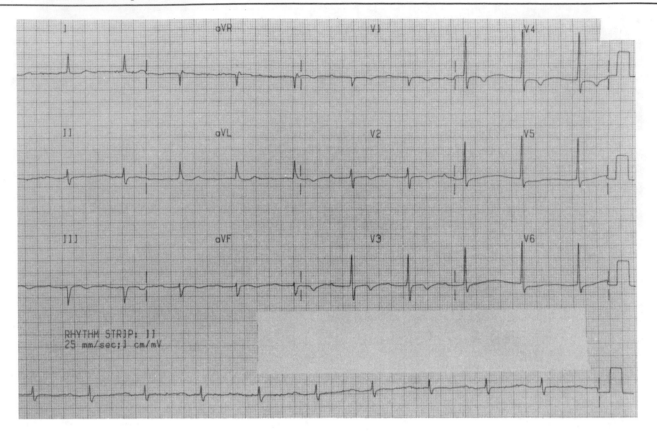

EKG 59

The P-R interval is .36 sec long.
1. At what point in the conduction pathway does this delay occur?
ANSWER: The P-R interval begins with the advance of the depolarization process from the S-A node and concludes with the onset of depolarization of the interventricular septum. Enroute, the process traverses the S-A–A-V tracts, the A-V node, the bundle of His, and the bundle branches. First-degree A-V block (prolonged P-R interval) may be caused by conduction delay in any of these segments, although the most common site lies in the A-V junctional tissue. In this patient, the duration of the P wave (.08 sec) and of the QRS complex (.08 sec) give reason to believe intra-atrial and bundle branch conduction are normal.

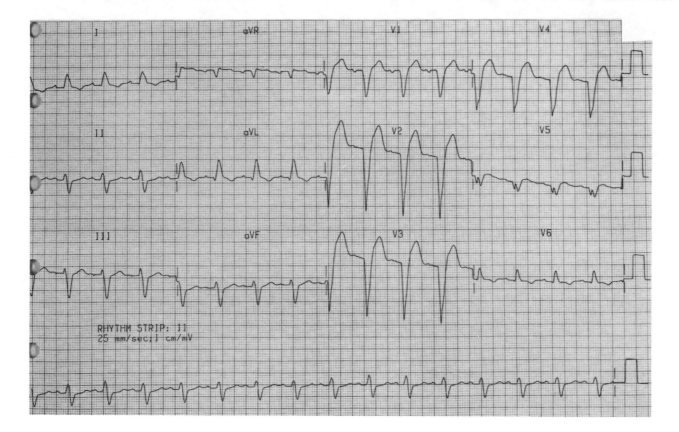

EKG 60

Although intraventricular conduction delay is the striking abnormality in this record, let us concern ourselves with the P waves here. The duration of P waves ranges from .10 to .12 sec in various leads. Normal limits of P-wave duration are considered to be .05 to .12 sec, and normal amplitude to be less than 2 mm (.2 mV). The P waves here are notable for the broad, notched configuration in leads V_2 through V_4 and the negative terminal portion in lead V_1. As discussed elsewhere, prominence of the latter half of the P wave is suggestive of left atrial enlargement or damage because the last portion of the atria to be depolarized is that region which is furthest from the S-A node. This record, therefore, suggests left atrial enlargement.

Left atrial enlargement is most frequently the result of increase in its "afterload" either because of mitral stenosis or of left ventricular disease.

Thus, if clinical evidence of mitral stenosis is not present, we can reasonably conclude that left ventricular damage has occurred with impairment in ventricular filling. In fact, this 78-year-old man had had coronary bypass and ventricular aneurysmectomy, and at the time of this record, presented evidence of left ventricular failure.

The intraventricular conduction delay should not be attributed to left bundle block because initial depolarization is from left to right. The Q waves in leads I, aVL, and V_6 and the QS segment in leads V_1 through V_5 are compatible with the echocardiographic demonstration of a dyskinetic septal infarction and widespread hypokinesis. Indeed, the precordial leads reveal encroachment of this lesion into the anterior lateral wall.

1. How should we classify the conduction delay?

ANSWER: Either as left anterior hemiblock or peri-infarction block. In this case, both terms are equally appropriate.

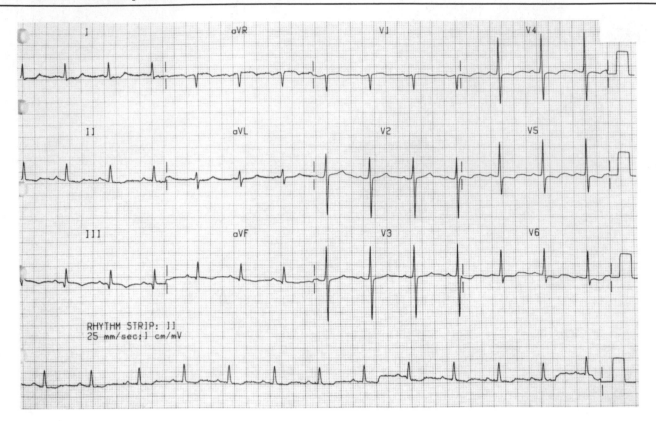

RHYTHM STRIP: II
25 mm/sec;1 cm/mV

EKG 61

1. Which of the 12 electrocardiographic leads is "most reliable"?

ANSWER: Each of the leads presents "reliable" information; however, lead I is the least subject to variation because of variations in electrical position and, therefore, is distorted less frequently by shifts in position.

Lead I will, to be sure, fail to produce evidence of any electrical disorder that is limited to the plane lying 90° to its axis. Thus, a directly anterior, posterior, or inferior abnormality will not be registered; however, an abnormality whose mean vector lies at an angle off that plane will produce a change in lead I.

Because this lead is not subject to "insignificant" variations, the S-T depression in lead I would have required our attention even if the remainder of the record had been normal (which it is not).

Lead III is the lead *most* frequently altered by physiologic and spatial variables. Because of its position in space, its 90° plane may lie almost

parallel with the initial septal vector and the apical vector. A slight positional change may, therefore, cause projections of these two vectors to vary from positive to negative or vice versa. The free-wall

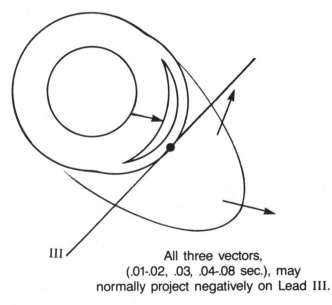

III

All three vectors,
(.01-.02, .03, .04-.08 sec.), may
normally project negatively on Lead III.

Case 61

.04- to .08-sec vector may readily cast a negative projection in lead III. Thus, Q waves of .01 to .03 sec and even QS waves as long as .08 sec may be registered in normal persons in this lead. A good rule is to test lead III by the findings in lead II and/or aVF. If those two leads appear normal, the appearance of Q or QS in lead III should be considered a normal variant (Case 61).

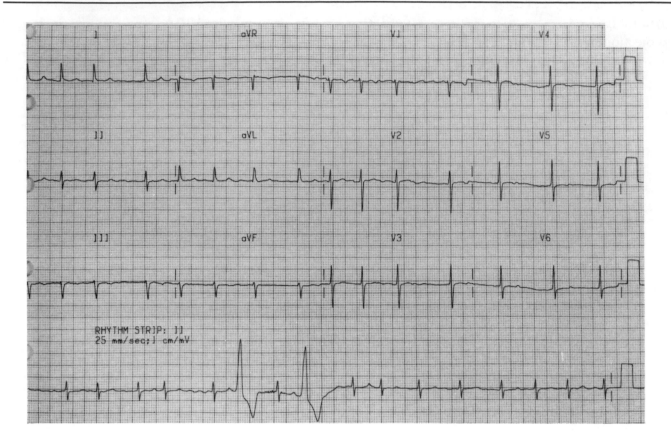

EKG 62

Lead V_1 is often especially useful in identifying atrial rhythm, apparently because the electrode lies in close proximity to the atria.

1. What is the rhythm here?

ANSWER: There is an old saying that if, on first glance, lead V_1 suggests flutter, the correct diagnosis may be fibrillation. The secret of proper interpretation lies in observation of a consistent repetitive atrial wave (flutter) versus irregular, constantly varying atrial waves (fibrillation). Often, by chance, fibrillation will produce a brief run of apparently regular atrial waves; however, this does not continue in a sustained, regular fashion.

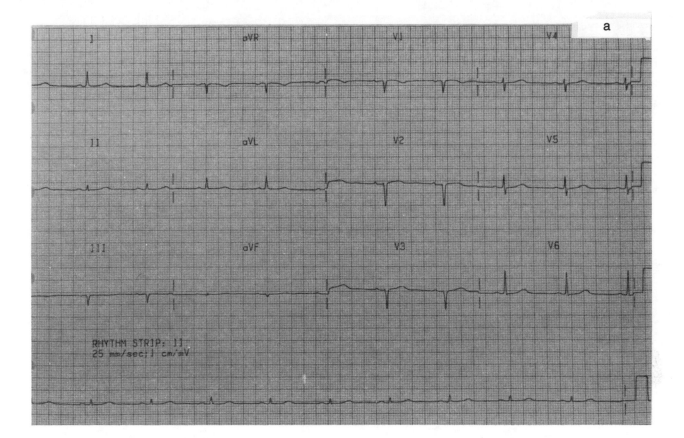

EKG 63

This configuration in the precordial leads is often seen in otherwise normal records and has been designated "clockwise rotation" or "poor progression of R waves." It is essential to recognize that "clockwise rotation" is a term that is *descriptive* of electrical manifestations but that does not *explain* their occurrence.

1. What possible variants could diminish the initial amplitude of the R wave of right and anterior precordial leads as seen in record 63a?

ANSWER: Simple rotation of the heart about its long axis might account for loss of septal vectors as they are projected on leads V_2, V_3 and V_4.

Other variants might equally well produce this phenomenon. If the position of the heart were shifted headward in relation to the electrodes in leads V_1 through V_3, septal depolarization would advance initially toward these electrodes, then pass beyond them and present a negative, trailing component of the dipole to these leads. Therefore, they might show a small r wave followed by a prominent S wave. Although clockwise rotation and headward shift of the position of the heart may alter the configuration of the V leads, poor progression of R waves or clockwise rotation are often seen without evidence of physical displacement of the heart. Other possibilities must be admitted.

If the initial "beachhead" of depolarization of the septum were located at midseptum or near the base of the septum rather than near the apex, septal depolarization would present a diminished positive or indeed a negative charge in leads V_1, V_2, and V_3 (see Fig. I-146).

If the initial beachhead on the septum were placed in an anterior position on the septum, the depolarization of the septum would advance predominantly in a posterior direction, and leads V_1 through V_3 would show a diminished early positive charge. If, on the other hand, the initial beachhead is on the posterior portion of the septum, its depolarization would advance toward those electrodes and

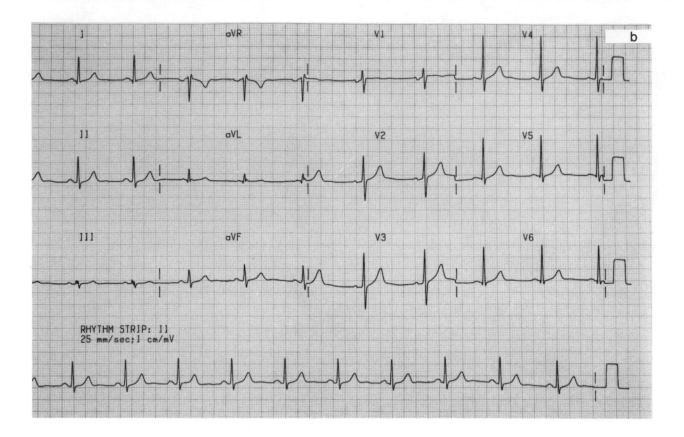

RHYTHM STRIP: II
25 mm/sec;1 cm/mV

would generate unusually prominent R waves in the right precordial leads ("counterclockwise rotation"), (Record 63b).

2. Record 63c presents another EKG with R waves of interest in leads V_1, V_2 and V_3. Could the reduction in size of the R wave in lead V_3 when compared with leads V_2 and V_1 be attributed to simple clockwise rotation?

ANSWER: No. The normal variants that have been mentioned do not produce a loss of R-wave amplitude in a V lead when compared with its predecessor. Thus the R wave in lead V_2 will not normally be smaller than it is in lead V_1, nor will the R wave in lead V_3 be less than the R in lead V_2. The explanation for the reduction of R-wave amplitude in lead V_3 in record 63c is obvious when one considers the abnormalities in leads II, III, and aVF. The abnormalities in those leads reveal evidence of a diaphragmatic myocardial infarction. The reduction in R-wave amplitude in lead V_3 almost certainly results from an anterior "arm" of the diaphragmatic infarction extending into the anterior ventricular wall, with sufficient loss of myocardial population to reduce R-wave height but without sufficient depopulation to generate a Q wave.

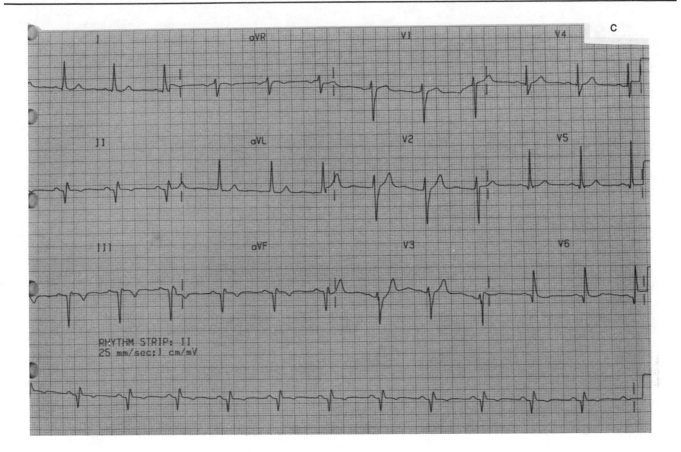

RHYTHM STRIP: II
25 mm/sec: 1 cm/mV

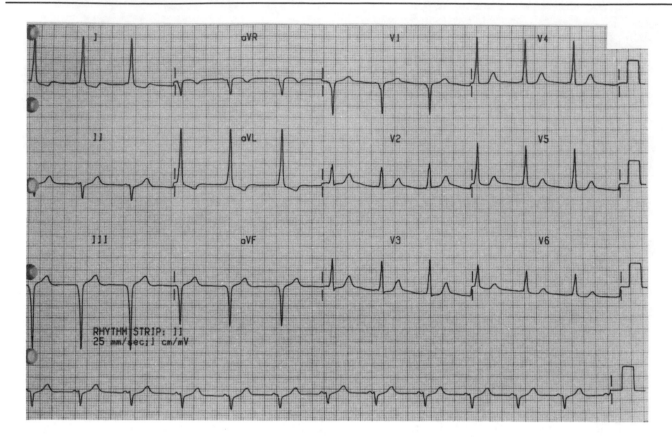

EKG 64

The large QS complex in leads III and aVF and the prominent R waves in leads V_2 through V_4 might suggest loss of diaphragmatic posterior myocardium. Such a conclusion would be a serious error.

1. What is the proper interpretation?

ANSWER: Pre-excitation syndrome (Wolff-Parkinson-White), in which the pre-excitation "bridge" between the atria and ventricles is so located as to prematurely activate an area at the base of the ventricles, is the correct explanation. This early "beachhead" produces depolarization dipoles that advance anteriorly and superiorly from the base of the right ventricle. The negative aspect of these dipoles generates negative delta waves in leads III and aVF and upright delta waves in leads V_2 through V_5. That these initial waves are delta waves and not pathologic Q waves in leads III and aVF is confirmed by the short P-R interval (.07 to .08 sec) and the prolonged QRS complex (.10 sec).

2. What do the S-T,T configurations mean here?

ANSWER: The S-T,T waves are normal in most of the leads because the predominant mass of the ventricles is depolarizing and repolarizing in a normal fashion. The pre-excited area, therefore, represents a minor portion of the heart. The S-T,T in leads I, aVL, and V_6 is deformed because the influence of the pre-excitation process is most powerfully directed toward those leads; thus, the *premature re*polarization of the pre-excited area is most apparent in those leads.

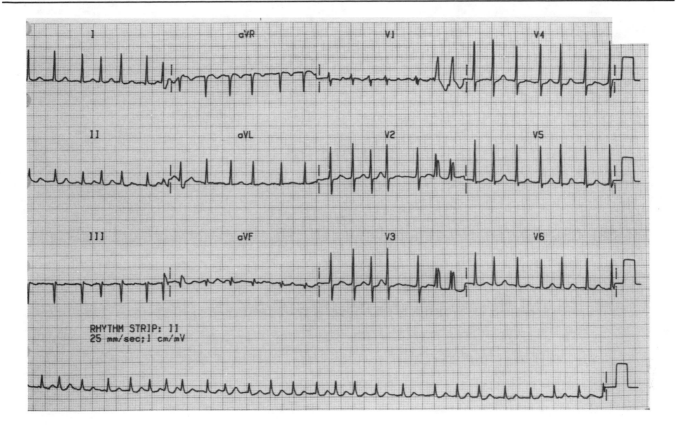

EKG 65

In the presence of rapid supraventricular rhythm, ventricular response varies from 145 to 190 beats per minute. The final beat in leads I, II, and III and the final two beats in leads V_1, V_2, and V_3 are notably different from the rest.

1. Are they premature ventricular contractions?

ANSWER: Note that the interval between these beats and their prodecessors is the shortest seen in the record, .260 to .280 sec. All other beats, even those with an interbeat interval as short as .300 sec have "normal" QRS configuration. These beats almost certainly, there-fore, represent aberrant intraventricular conduction. When the interbeat interval is less than .280 sec in this case, some portion of the right bundle branch system remains refrac-tory, and the resulting depolarization has an incomplete right bundle branch block config-uration. The distinction between this phe-nomenon (Ashman phenomenon) and premature ventricular contractions lies in rec-ognition of the fact that this phenomenon oc-curs after an exceptionally short interbeat interval.

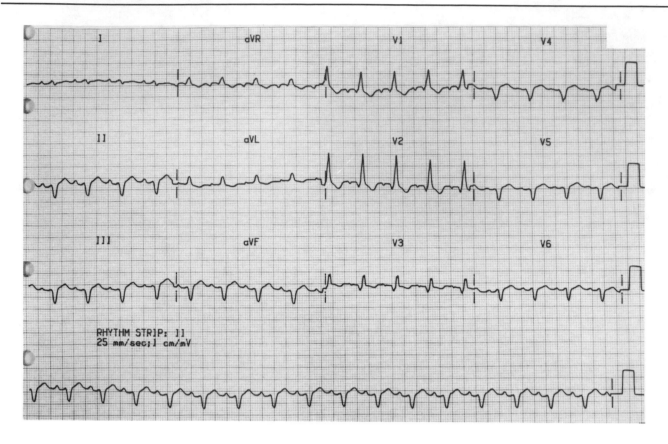

EKG 66

Right bundle branch block and left anterior hemiblock are seen here.

1. Does the record indicate anything else?

ANSWER: In right bundle branch block, the QRS configuration in leads V_1 and V_2 and often in V_3 is an rSR' or rSRs, the initial r representing septal depolarization. The absence of that r wave here indicates absence of septal depolarization, which in turn, implies absence of electrically active septal myocardium. Because death of myocardium is most often the result of ischemic infarction, this record is most indicative of anteroseptal necrosis (of unknown duration). Perhaps we should remind ourselves that pathologic Q waves mean loss of electrically active tissue; but it is an *assumption* based on the relative frequency of diseases, when we, without other data, attribute the Q wave to ischemic infarction.

Tumor, focal myocarditis, and trauma are some of the other potential causes of pathologic Q waves.

2. What is the geographic extent of the lesion here?

ANSWER: The area of missing tissue, in addition to the anteroseptal myocardium, includes the anterior wall.

The diminutive R waves in lead V_6 are attributable, in part at least, to left anterior hemiblock. As you recall, depolarization of the anterior and lateral left ventricular walls in left anterior hemiblock moves in a circumferential and an apex-to-base direction rather than in the sun-burst fashion of normal hearts. Thus, the dipoles do not "face" leads V_3, V_4, and V_5 in anterior hemiblock as they do normally, but instead move "across" the viewing positions of those leads with resultant smaller-than-normal R waves followed by terminal S waves.

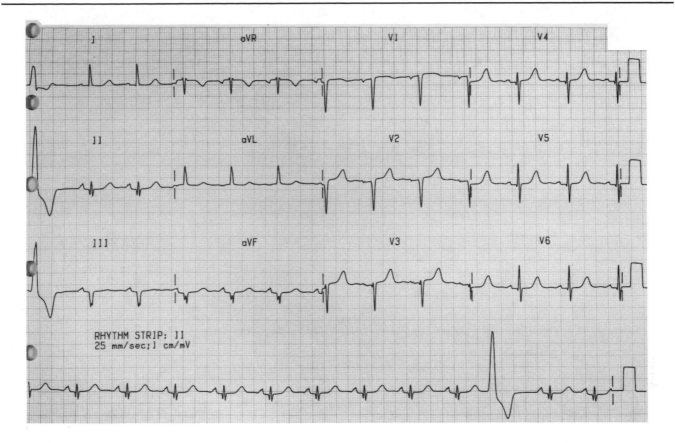

RHYTHM STRIP: II
25 mm/sec;1 cm/mV

EKG 67

In this record, there is an rS wave in lead V_1 followed by a QS segment in V_2.

1. How does one distinguish between a normal record with clockwise rotation and an anteroseptal infarction?

ANSWER: Usually, clockwise rotation in an otherwise normal record causes QS or rS waves in lead V_1 and rS in leads V_2 through V_4, but it will almost never cause the loss of r-wave amplitude in a succeeding lead. In this case, rS in lead V_1 is followed by a loss of r wave in V_2, and therefore, indicates a loss of depolarizing dipole in a segment of the anteroseptal myocardium.

2. Does the configuration of leads II, III, and aVF help interpret V_1, V_2, and V_3 here?

ANSWER: Yes. The QS in lead aVF is compatible with diaphragmatic infarction and therefore increases the possibility of ischemic lesions elsewhere.

3. Do the Q waves in leads V_3 through V_6 help one to recognize infarction?

ANSWER: No. These are normal .01- to .02-sec Q waves. In fact, their presence indicates survival of some portion of the septum.

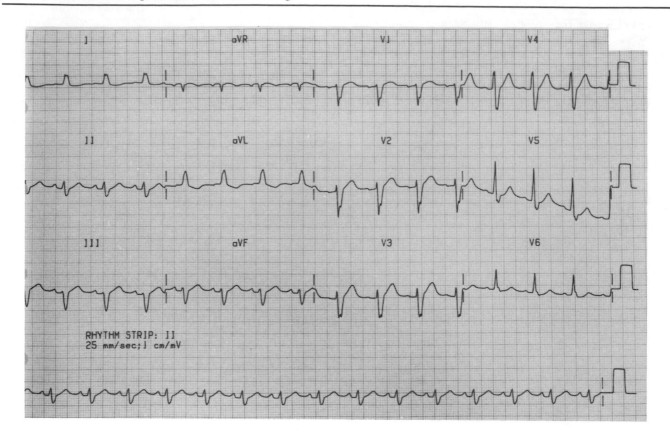

RHYTHM STRIP: II
25 mm/sec; 1 cm/mV

EKG 68

Left bundle branch block is seen here. Let us direct our attention to the S waves and R waves.

1. What accounts for the R waves in leads V_1, V_2, and V_3 if the septum is depolarized from right to left in left bundle branch block?

ANSWER: Depolarization of the right ventricular free wall occurs "on time" in this situation and contributes an anterior and rightward vector. Simultaneously, the septum is depolarized from the right bundle "beachhead." The process advances across the septum, toward the base and apex, and circumferentially into the posterior and anterior walls of the left ventricle. The positive waves in leads V_1 through V_3 here are the sum of these vectors. A posterior position of the septal "beachhead", or horizontal heart position with advance of dipoles up the septum toward leads V_1 and V_2 would provide positive projection of septal depolarization on these leads.

2. From leads V_2 through V_5, the R wave grows taller and its duration is greater. What does this mean?

ANSWER: As the recording electrodes lie further to the left, they face more directly the left side of the septum and of the free wall. The vectors generated are therefore more powerfully projected on the more leftward leads. The increasing duration of the R waves results from the increasing contribution of the later-to-depolarize free wall.

3. Why is the R wave smaller in lead V_6 than in lead V_5?

ANSWER: There is more air-filled lung between lead V_6 (midaxillary line) and the heart than between leads V_4 and V_5 (near the point of maximum impulse) and the heart. This "insulation" may diminish the R wave, and may contribute to the smaller amplitude of the S and T waves in lead V_6 in this record.

4. Why are the T waves tall in leads V_1 through V_5 in this record? Would you not expect the left bundle block to delay depolarization and repolarization over the left heart?

ANSWER: In this record, the area of maximum delay lies posteriorly, superiorly, and laterally, as indicated by the S waves in lead aVF and the V leads. Thus, the anterior as well as the right region will repolarize first. One might simplistically visualize the cone-shaped heart lying with its apex pointing nearly horizontally to the left while it is rotated on its long axis so as to direct its left wall superiorly and posteriorly.

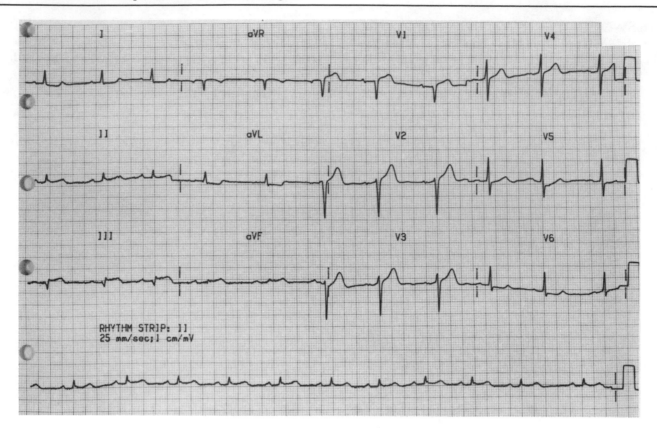

RHYTHM STRIP: II
25 mm/sec; 1 cm/mV

EKG 69

Downward S-T deviations in leads I, aVL, and V$_5$ and V$_6$, and S-T elevations in leads II, III, and aVF are present.

1. Are they diagnostic?

ANSWER: Yes. The deviation of the entire length of the S-T segment, the nearly horizontal slope of the S-T, and the reciprocal deviations are important indicators of acute myocardial injury. Because severe ischemic injury leads to loss of normal resting potential, a diastolic dipole is generated by severe injury (page 28). Because this dipole elevates or depresses the base line of the record, except when that dipole is extinguished by depolarization of the ventricles (the S-T segment), the S-T segment in this situation is the only portion of the ventricular complex that lies on "true zero" and is therefore a *horizontal* line identical with true zero.

2. How would one distinguish this record from a normal variant with so-called premature repolarization?

ANSWER: In that phenomenon, the S-T elevation is concave upward and typically ends in a prominently upright T wave. Its mechanism was discussed on pages 60 to 63.

3. Could this record be due to pericarditis?

ANSWER: Pericarditis is almost always a widespread epicardial process with all leads except aVR facing the subepicardial population of damaged cells. Therefore, all leads except aVR (which faces the endocardium) reveal S-T elevation. In addition, P-R depression (page 59) may be a diagnostically helpful manifestation of pericarditis.

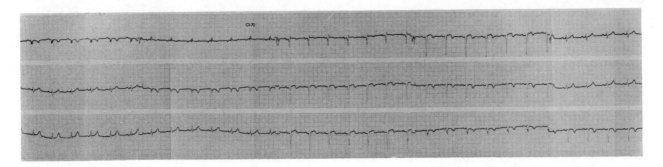

EKG 70

This record shows evidence of an extensive anterior myocardial infarction. The infarction occurred in December, 1983. This record was recorded in February, 1986.

1. In view of the electrocardiographic abnormalities, would you expect the patient has been (a) a cardiac invalid, (b) moderately limited by his cardiac disease, or (c) an active person?

ANSWER: During the interval between 1983 and 1986, the patient has been active and asymptomatic. This record illustrates that the development of the pathologic QS or the pathologic reduction in R-wave amplitude does not indicate *total* loss of myocardial cell population. Instead, it indicates loss of cell numbers sufficient to cause the cell population of the opposite healthy wall to exceed that in the damaged wall underlying the exploring electrodes. This patient resembles many others who have retained sufficient ventricular contractile function to lead active lives despite extensive QS evidence of myocardial loss.

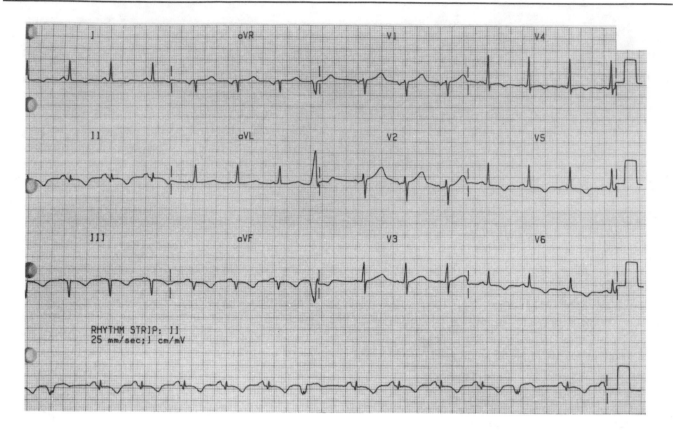

RHYTHM STRIP: II
25 mm/sec; 1 cm/mV

EKG 71

Often, an array of clinical information can be derived from the EKG.

1. List the possibilities you might consider after reviewing this record.

ANSWER: The patient has had a diaphragmatic myocardial infarction.

1. Without an S-T shift, the record does not indicate an active process. Comparison with other records would be necessary to exclude that possibility, because this record could have been made at a time in the evolution of a recent infarction in which the S-T segments have returned to isoelectric position.

2. The arterial lesion probably lies in the right coronary artery because that vessel most frequently supplies the diaphragmatic posterior myocardium. Less frequently, the posterior descending extension of the left circumflex artery is the nutrient vessel for that region.

3. The area of ischemic damage extends into the anterior and lateral wall of the left ven-

tricle. Either some loss of cells or sarcolemmal dysfunction of cells has occurred in this segment, but there has not been en-bloc destruction of the myocardium of the anterior and lateral walls. The vascular lesion responsible may be a branch of the anterior descending artery or of the circumflex vessel. On occasion, with right coronary dominance, this anterior lateral region may derive its blood supply from the right. The odds are, however, that this patient is afflicted with two- or three-vessel disease.

4. The large, notched P waves indicate left atrial enlargement. In turn, in the absence of mitral stenosis, this implies left ventricular dysfunction (in this case, either loss of compliance or loss of contractile function). Therefore, the P wave here is an indicator of abnormal left ventricular hemodynamic performance. The signs of left ventricular hypertrophy or left ventricular strain are not present. We must acknowledge that their absence does not exclude the possibility of left ventricular

hypertrophy. The classic QRS, S-T,T configuration is a highly specific, but only moderately sensitive, indicator of left ventricular hypertrophy. In one autopsy series, approximately 20% of those with confirmed left ventricular hypertrophy had presented this classic EKG configuration. In approximately 40% of those studied, only the S-T,T evidence of left ventricular strain had been present. The approximately 40% remaining had other abnormalities, such as bundle block or infarction, but no sign of hypertrophy or strain had appeared on EKG. Premature ventricular contractions with Qr in lead aVF, QS in lead II, and Rs in lead aVL suggest the premature contractions probably originate in the inferior wall and advance headward. Thus, they may arise in or near the diaphragmatic infarction. The possibility of one-way conduction from a focus adjacent to a poorly conducting infarct, and with it, the possibility of reentry ventricular arrhythmia should come to mind on viewing this record.

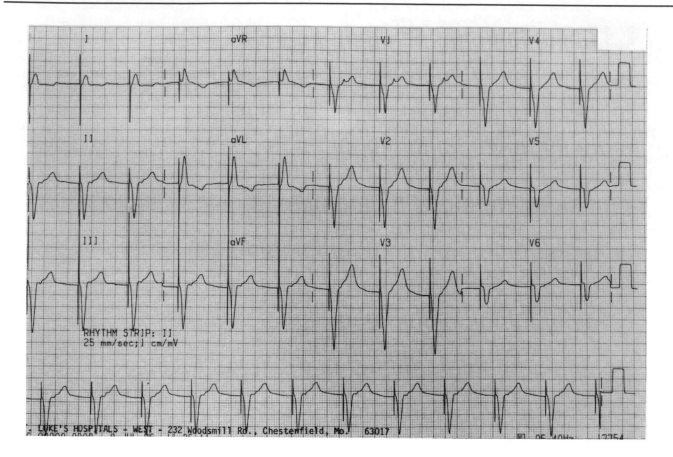

RHYTHM STRIP: II
25 mm/sec; 1 cm/mV

LUKE'S HOSPITALS - WEST - 232 Woodsmill Rd., Chesterfield, Mo.   63017

EKG 72

1. What was the indication for pacemaker installation here?

ANSWER: Probably sick sinus syndrome or another bradyarrhythmia. Because the pacemaker depolarizations of the ventricles are conducted retrograde into the atria (note the retrograde P waves in the S-T segments of leads V_1, V_2, II, III, and aVF), it is unlikely (*but not impossible*) that the pacemaker was required because of A-V block.

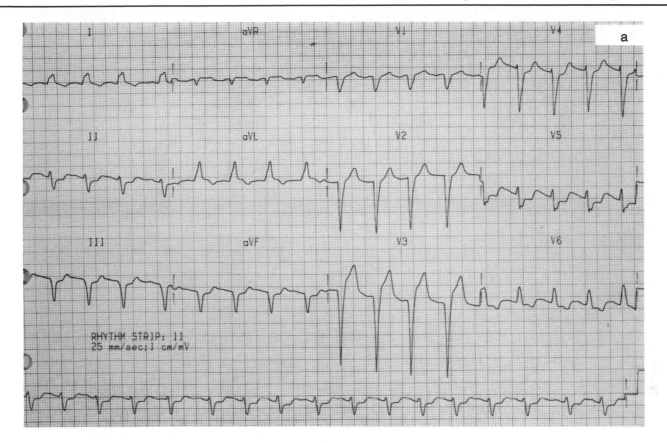

RHYTHM STRIP: II
25 mm/sec;1 cm/mV

EKG 73

This patient, a 77-year-old woman, suffered severe unstable angina. During coronary angiography, it was discovered that she had total occlusion of the right coronary artery, 50% obstruction of the left main coronary artery, 90% obstruction of the left anterior descending artery and of the circumflex coronary artery. During her hospital course, several electrocardiograms were recorded. Each of them revealed left bundle branch block.

1. What is the significance of the S-T,T variations seen in this series of records?

ANSWER: Records 73b and 73c show S-T,T features that one might readily attribute to the left bundle branch block itself. Record 73a shows new S-T abnormalities, with S-T depression most evident in leads V_5, II, and aVF and reciprocal S-T elevation in leads I, aVL, and V_3. These nearly horizontal S-T deviations are compatible with a regional abnormality of myocardial cellular membranes so severe as to produce a regional reduction of resting potential. This series illustrates that S-T,T abnormalities can be clinically important even in the presence of left bundle branch block. Granted, horizontal S-T depressions may be the result of left bundle branch block when phase 2 of the action potential is downsloping, as illustrated on pages 99 to 100. When, however, *fluctuations* of S-T,T configuration of the magnitude seen in this record develop without further alteration in conduction delay, the change can be virtually diagnostic of fresh myocardial injury.

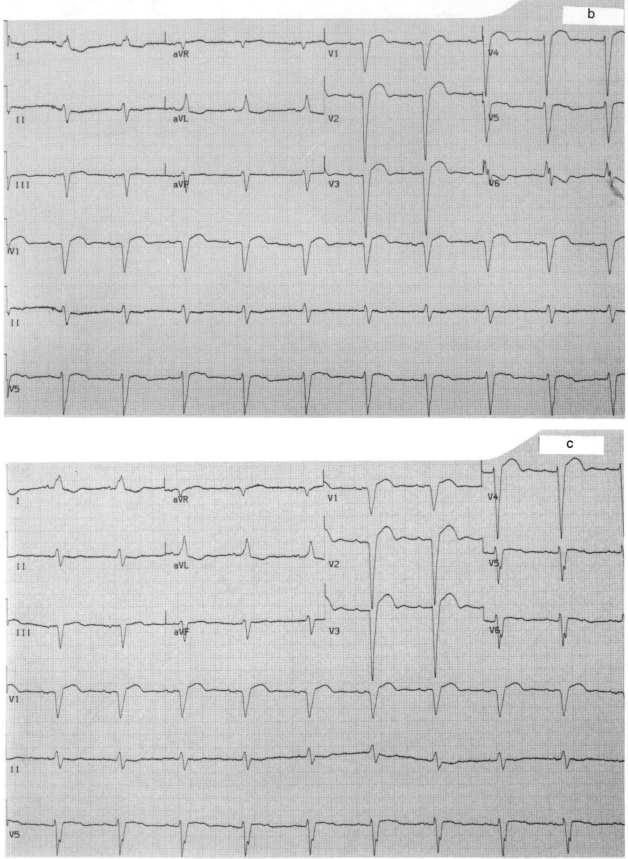

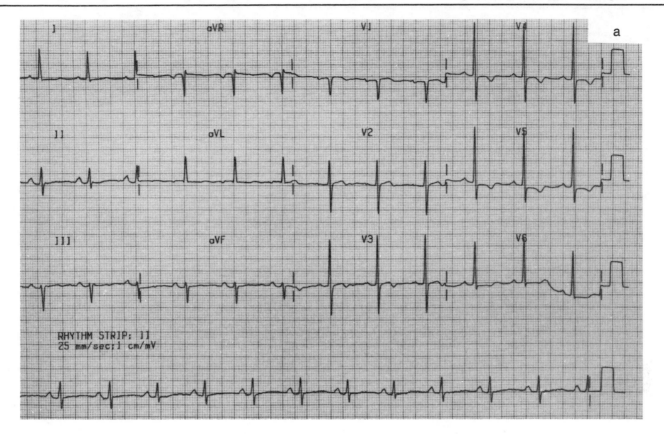

RHYTHM STRIP: II
25 mm/sec; 1 cm/mV

EKG 74

This series of electrocardiograms, recorded over a 10-day period, might serve as a biography of the patient.

1. What basic processes do the S-T,T variations suggest? What clinical events might be responsible?

ANSWER: The inverted T waves in leads V_3 through V_6 on day 1 (records 74a and b) and day 3 (74c) are compatible with cellular damage productive of either (a) *shortening* of the action potential of anterior and lateral *subendocardial* myocardial cells or (b) *lengthening* of the action potential of the whole *transmural* array of anterior and lateral myocardial cells. In either case, the repolarization process would present a negative net charge to leads V_3 through V_6.

2. On day 4 (record d), the T waves became upright in leads V_3 through V_6 and in leads II, III, and aVF. Is this good news or bad news?

ANSWER: Such an abrupt change to "normal" often reflects *new* damage, because acute fresh cellular insult may so alter sarcolemmal in-

tegrity as to hasten the leak of potassium from cells during phase 3 and thus accelerate repolarization of the injured cells. The T waves may be *freshly* upright or impressively tall in leads overlying the lesion because these cells are repolarizing more rapidly than their more normal mates. Another factor that may account for the hyperacute change of T waves is the ischemic release of catecholamines from the sympathetic nerve endings in the area of acute insult. The sympathomimetic hastening of repolarization facilitates premature development of positive surface charges around these ischemic cells and thereby generates positive T waves in the overlying leads.

Abrupt *improvement* of the myocardium *might* have occurred on day 4 (74d); however, the rapidity of the change should make one cautious about this interpretation until subsequent records confirm sustained improvement.

In this patient, records made later on day 4 and on days 5 and 6 (74e, 74f, and 74g) revealed recurrence of T-wave inversions as

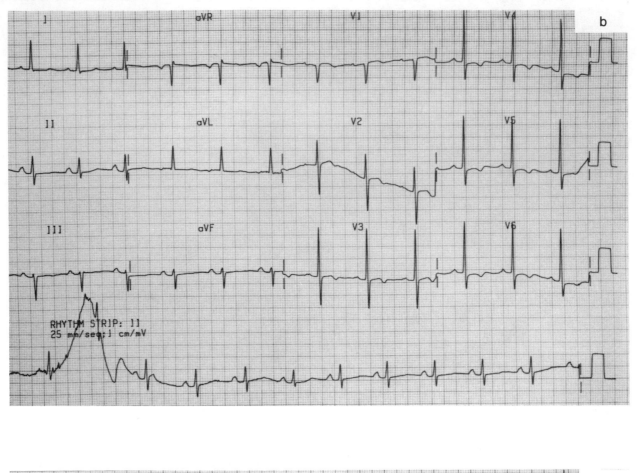

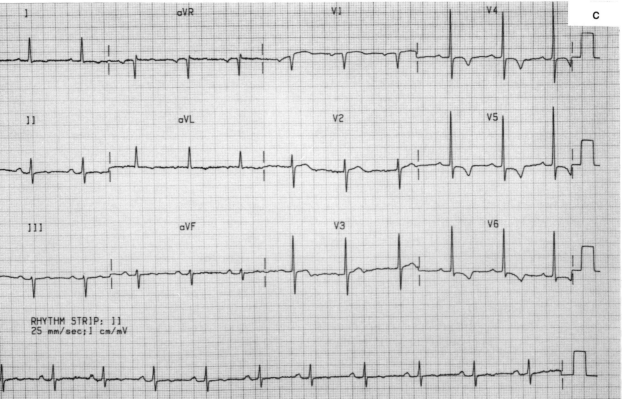

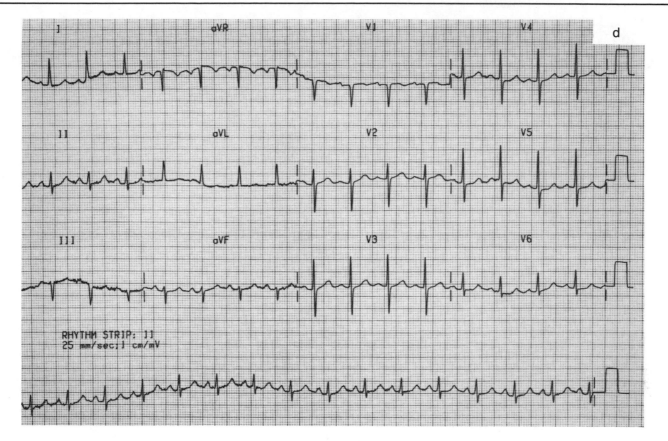

though the ischemic state had returned to what it had been prior to day 4.

Finally, on day 10 (74h) the S-T,T configuration evolved toward normal in a fashion commonly seen in recovery from an ischemic episode.

This patient, a 77-year-old woman, was admitted with recurrent episodes of left anterior and left shoulder pain. Enzyme analyses done in proper sequence revealed normal CK and CK-MB (creatine kinase-MB). The series of electrocardiograms was compatible with a fluctuating state of myocardial ischemia that never became so severe as to cause cell death or dysfunction sufficient to alter the resting potential. As has been stated, myocardial cells are analogous to boats with built-in leaks and built-in bailing apparatus designed to keep their "bottoms" dry. In this case, the sarcolemmal pumps manage to keep the "boats" dry (normal resting potential) despite damage to the membrane "bailers."

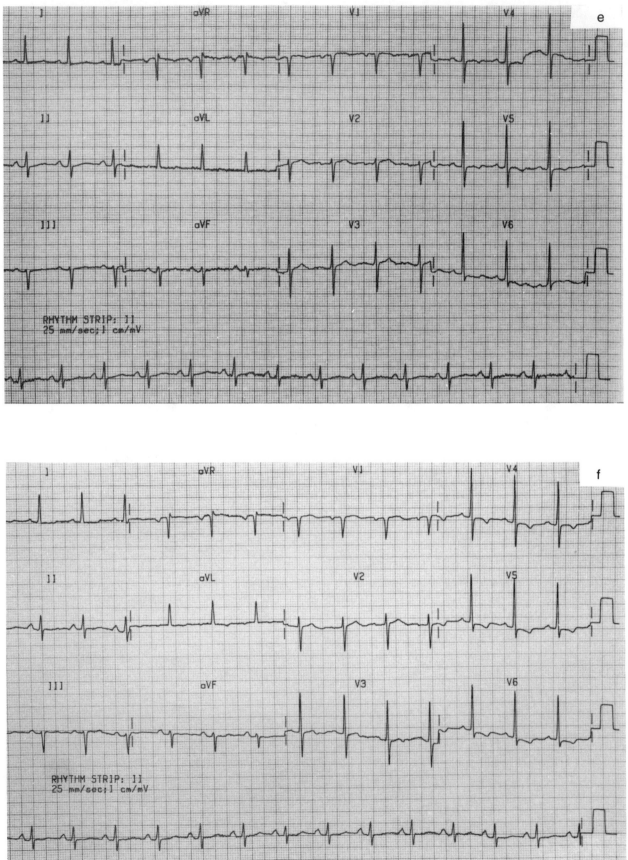

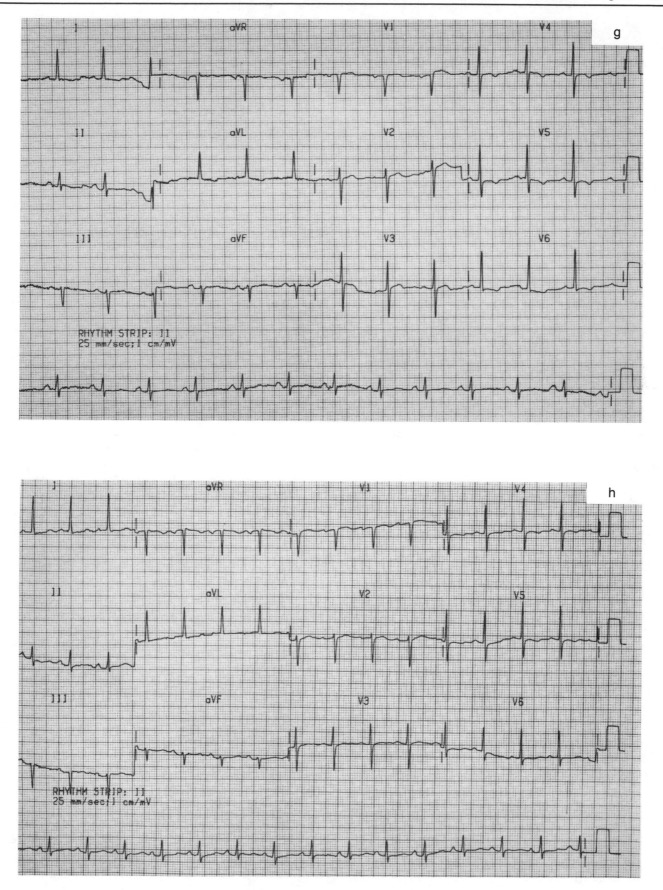

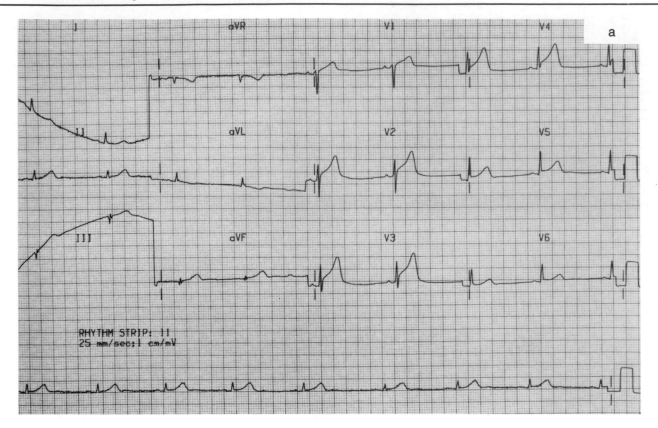

EKG 75

EKG 75a was recorded immediately after the patient was admitted to the hospital.

1. What is the significance of the S-T,T configuration?

ANSWER: Occasionally, impressive S-T elevations and tall T waves may be normal variants (page 60). Supporting clinical data and unchanging serial records would be required before one could accept this as a benign normal variant. In this instance, the second tracing recorded 3 hours later in the cardiac catheterization laboratory indicates the true nature of this patient's problem.

2. What are the processes revealed by this pair of electrocardiograms?

ANSWER: The loss of R waves from leads V_1 through V_3 and the partial loss of R waves from leads V_4 through V_6 indicate loss of sarcolemmal depolarization and imply severe sarcolemmal damage or death. The S-T,T configurations in the first record represent the early stages of the ischemic process before cellular death.

3. Does this mean all cells underlying leads V_1 through V_3 have ceased to function?

ANSWER: No. With the development of the QS in leads V_1 through V_3, one can know that the functioning cell population in the anteroseptal anterior wall has become *less* than the population of the *opposite* ventricular wall. As discussed on page 26, normally the cell population depolarizing toward anterior and lateral leads exceeds that facing the opposite direction because of the horseshoe shape of the left ventricle. That a pathologic QS does not mean total loss of cells is often demonstrated by echocardiographic studies, which commonly show residual albeit subnormal contractile motion in the involved area.

4. How can one quantitate the loss of cells in this situation?

ANSWER: The depth of the QS is roughly proportional to the ratio of cell populations in the affected and opposite walls. Thus, either increased cell loss in the affected myocardium or hypertrophy of the opposite wall will magnify the QS in leads overlying an infarct.

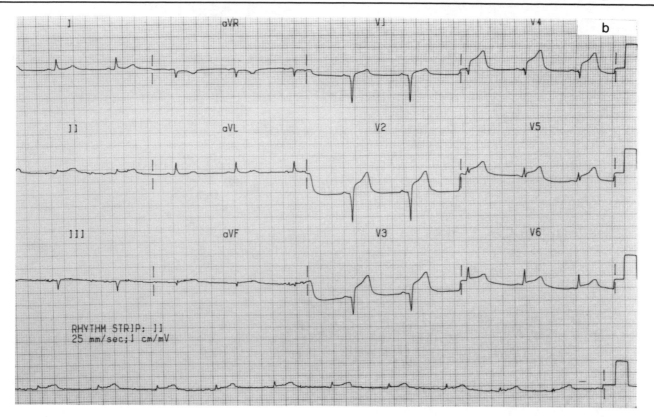

5. What is the significance of the diminution of R waves in leads V_4 through V_6?

ANSWER: The intensity of depopulation decreases as one advances from "ground zero" of the infarction to its periphery.

6. Does the absence of Q waves in leads I, aVL, and V_4 through V_6 deserve comment?

ANSWER: Yes. The absence of the normal septal Q wave is the result of septal cellular depletion.

   EKG 75b, recorded a few hours after 75a, presents large QS waves indicative of cellular death. Despite this major change, little if any further alteration in S-T,T occurred.

7. How can this be?

ANSWER: These records illustrate a fundamental point: Loss of R waves and development of QS waves result from arrest of sarcolemmal function usually as a result of cellular death, whereas these S-T,T abnormalities represent sarcolemmal dysfunction of damaged but still living cells. Between the recording of 75a and 75b, a number of myocardial cells died, but a large population of casualties survived. The tall T waves seen in 75a and 75b may represent the hyperacute T-wave phenomenon that has been discussed. The persistently upright T wave recorded 24 hours later in 75c cannot, however, be related to the release of catecholamines from ischemic intramyocardial nerve endings because that process is not likely to persist for so many hours; instead, the tall T waves can be attributed to persistent acceleration of repolarization of the ischemic cells (page 125). The T-wave height is further magnified by displacement of the baseline downward by loss of resting potential of the severely damaged cells. In record 75d, the nadir of the final portion of the T waves in precordial leads was positioned well below the S-T segment. *Had the baseline been isoelectric and the resultant illusion of S-T elevation abolished, the T waves in this record would have been 5 mm deep in leads V_2 and V_3, 2 to 4 mm deep in leads V_4 and V_5, and 1 mm deep in lead V_6.*

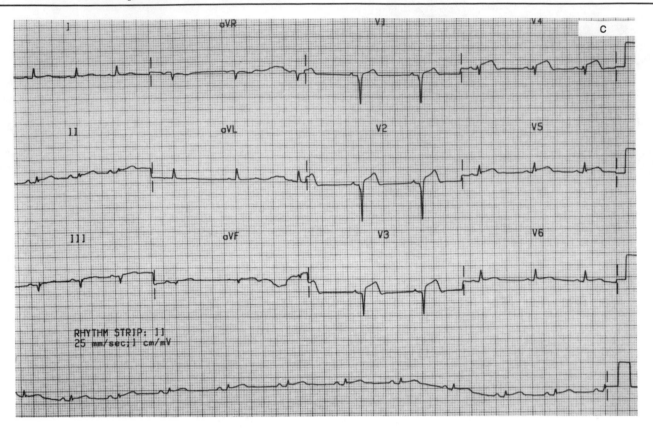

A second factor in the progressive T-wave inversion in this series of records is almost certainly the progressive death of cells in the infarcted area with an increasing deficit in repolarizing dipoles within the lesion. Thus, the abnormality of the ratio of repolarizing dipoles in the affected area to the dipoles in the opposite wall becomes more marked with the passage of time.

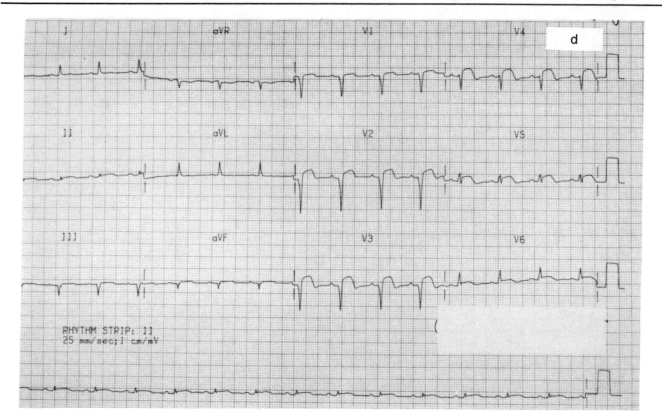

RHYTHM STRIP: II
25 mm/sec; 1 cm/mV

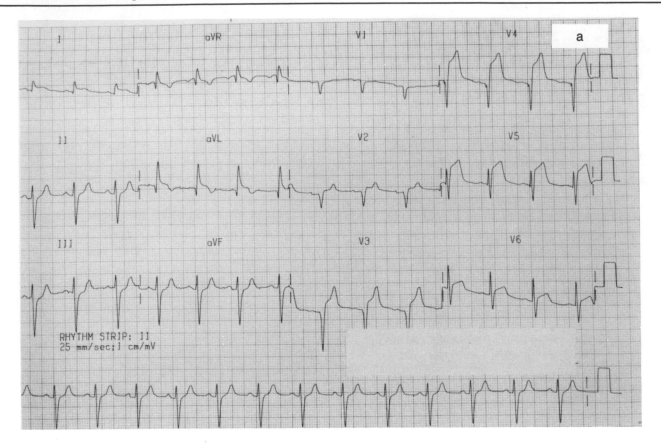

EKG 76

This series of records presents convincing evidence of an anteroseptal, anterior loss of sarcolemmal depolarization, regional loss of resting potential, and T waves compatible with an acute active disturbance of sarcolemmal repolarization: the constellation of abnormalities seen in infarction. The first record (76a) presented evidence of left anterior hemiblock. The second record (76b), taken after transfer to the coronary care unit from the emergency room, showed evidence of an additional intraventricular conduction problem.

1. What are the features diagnostic of left anterior hemiblock?

ANSWER: Left anterior hemiblock can be recognized when (1) left-axis deviation greater than −30°, (2) significant clockwise rotation (poor R wave progression), and (3) retention of normal septal Q wave co-exist. QRS duration may remain within normal limits or may be slightly prolonged.

2. What additional conduction defect appeared in record 76b?

ANSWER: The duration of the QRS increased from .10 sec to .13 sec with the development of late R waves in leads V_2 and V_3 without S waves in lead I or increased S waves in leads V_4 through V_6. This may represent right bundle branch block; most interpretors would probably draw that conclusion. An alternative explanation comes to mind, however, in view of the absence of the expected S waves in left lateral leads and the absence of R-R' or QR' in lead V_1. Delayed intraventricular conduction appears to be oriented directly forward (anteriorly) with tall, late R waves in leads V_2 and V_3. The problem, therefore, may be a peri-infarction block within the septum. Two days later, S waves have appeared in lead I and have become larger in leads V_4 through V_6. One cannot deny the presence of right bundle branch block (76c).

This patient was subjected to cardiac catheterization immediately following the development of an acute myocardial infarction. That study revealed significant hypokinesis of the apical seg-

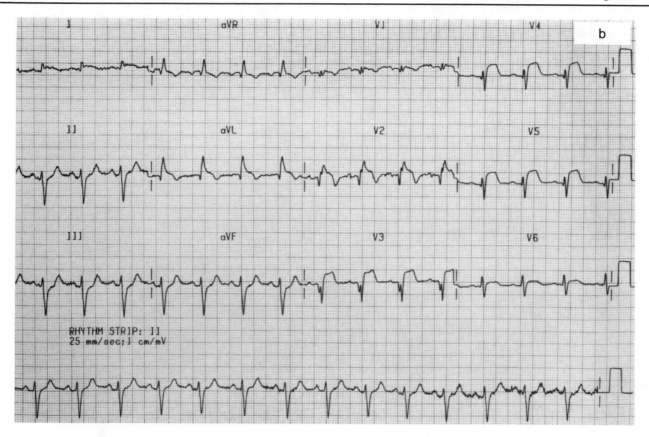

ment and adjoining parts of the inferior and anterior walls of the left ventricle. Strikingly, the proximal parts of both the anterior and inferior walls of the left ventricle showed reasonably healthy wall motion. This patient was found to have 70% obstruction of the right, 90% obstruction of the posterior descending, and 100% obstruction of the left anterior descending coronary arteries.

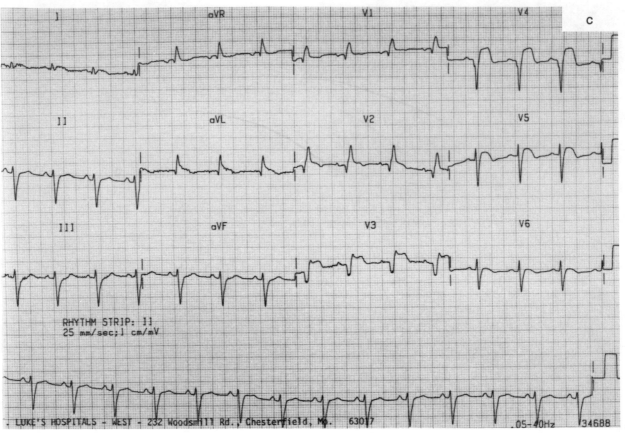

RHYTHM STRIP: II
25 mm/sec; 1 cm/mV

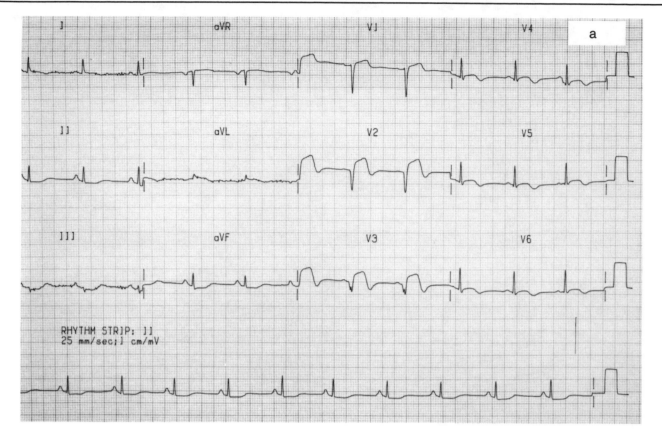

RHYTHM STRIP: II
25 mm/sec; 1 cm/mV

EKG 77

These tracings were recorded 2 days apart.

1. What is the primary electrocardiographic diagnosis?

ANSWER: The records indicate an anteroseptal anterior infarction with anterolateral ischemic injury.

2. How would you account for the changes between the first and second records? Has the patient experienced an uneventful post-infarction course or have there been complications?

ANSWER: The rapid return of upright T waves and the increased S-T elevations in leads V_3 through V_5 indicate fresh cellular damage between the first and second record (48-hour interval).

3. Is this a recurrent ischemic insult or is the new process pericarditis overlying infarction?

ANSWER: Either process is possible. The fact that reciprocal S-T depression did not occur in leads aVF, II, and III does not help us, because recurrent injury located directly ante-riorly would not provoke a reciprocal depression in inferior leads II, III, and aVF.

4. What is the significance of the findings in leads I and aVL in these records?

ANSWER: The small R waves and the S-T elevations indicate encroachment of the ischemic process on the lateral wall.

5. The peaked P waves are more noticeable on record 77b than on 77a. What could this signify?

ANSWER: This far-from-diagnostic change suggests right atrial enlargement. In turn, this raises the possibility of right ventricular dysfunction secondary to infarction of the right ventricle.

This patient, a 77-year-old man, was admitted to the hospital with severe chest pain. Serial CK-MB concentrations were indicative of acute myocardial infarction. Cardiac catheterization and coronary angiography revealed multivessel obstruction: 50% of the left main, 95% of the left anterior descending, 90% and 70% of the first and second diagonal, respectively, 90% of the circum-

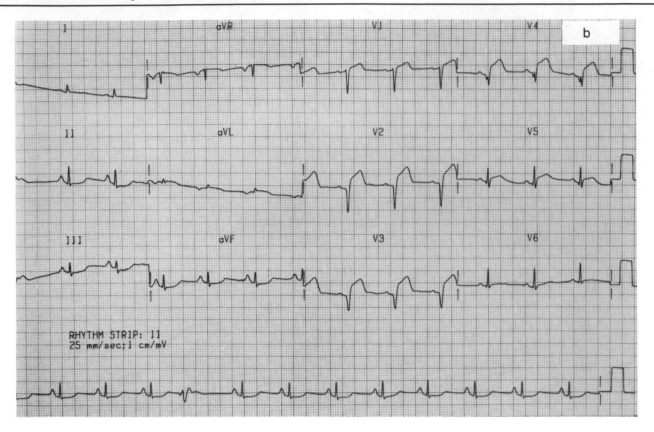

RHYTHM STRIP: II
25 mm/sec; 1 cm/mV

flex, 50% of the first marginal, and 70% of the right coronary arteries. Anterolateral and apical dyskinesis and global hypokinesis were observed. The electrocardiographic and angiographic evidence of anteroseptal, anterior, and lateral ischemic damage is obvious. One might question the meaning of the S-T segment depression in lead aVF. It may be the reciprocal effect of the anterior and lateral process, or it may instead reflect inferior subendocardial injury related to the 70% obstruction of the right coronary artery.

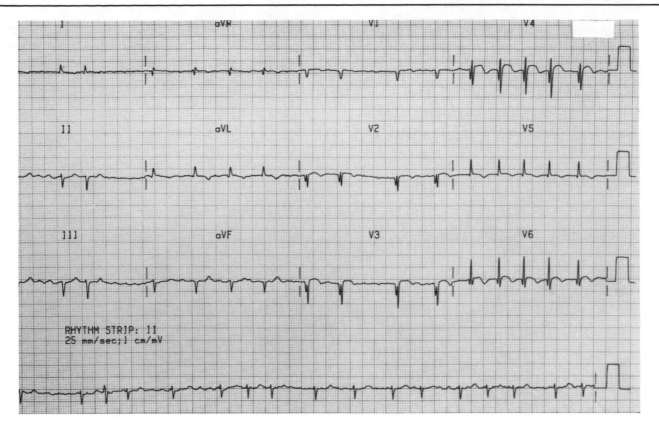

RHYTHM STRIP: II
25 mm/sec; 1 cm/mV

EKG 78

1. This anteroseptal anterior infarction is complicated by what condition(s)?

ANSWER: (1) Left anterior hemiblock. It is easy to visualize the interruption of anterior hemibranches because they lie across the area of septal infarction.

(2) Atrial fibrillation with intervals between ventricular contractions as long as .96 sec.

2. How does one account for the ventricular rate when hundreds of atrial depolarizations are "knocking on the door" of the A-V node per minute?

ANSWER: The broad-faced A-V node tapering into the bundle of His appears to be a filter-funnel designed to facilitate the collision of depolarizations entering through the multiple portals of entry of the node (see concealed conduction, page 83). The normal A-V node may be likened to a complex network of pathways converging onto a narrow bridge. Although this would be a highway engineer's nightmare, it is a highly effective means of blocking excessive traffic over the A-V bridge.

The functional importance of the *broad-face* of the nodal funnel can be appreciated when one considers how the situation is altered by a *narrow* A-V bridge, as seen in the pre-excitation syndrome. There, without collisions of impulses arriving through multiple portals, the frequency of A-V transmission is limited only by the duration of the refractory period of the A-V nodal pathway. Atrial fibrillation in patients with this condition may produce ventricular rates as high as 250 to 300 beats per minute. Excessively rapid ventricular response in the presence of atrial fibrillation should always bring to mind the possibility of such an accessory pathway.

In this patient, the prolonged .96-sec R-R interval may represent ischemic impairment of conduction over the A-V bridge.

This 65-year-old man came to the hospital because he had had chest pain for 24 hours. His serial electrocardiograms were compatible with an active or recent myocardial infarction. Properly timed enzyme measurements, however, failed to detect infarction.

3. What is the most likely explanation for the *discrepancy between the result of enzyme tests and EKGs* in this instance?

ANSWER: In all probability, this patient suffered a necrotic insult earlier and the serial enzyme measurements "missed" the rise and fall of MBs.

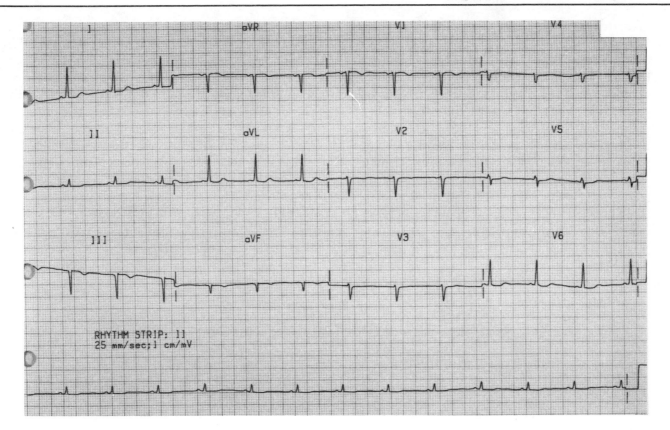

RHYTHM STRIP: II
25 mm/sec; 1 cm/mV

EKG 79

1. What are the notable features in this record?

ANSWER: (1) Diaphragmatic myocardial infarction.

(2) Nonspecific S-T,T configurations in leads I and V_6 compatible with left ventricular strain and/or digitalis effect.

(3) Poor progression of R waves in precordial leads (clockwise rotation). Such poor progression is one of the two components of left anterior hemiblock.

2. Does this patient have that problem?

ANSWER: No. The absence of left-axis deviation excludes that possibility.

Whereas both diaphragmatic infarction and left anterior hemiblock may produce left-axis deviation, the distinction between the two rests on the presence of an initial R wave in lead aVF in hemiblock and the absence of such an initial R wave in the presence of diaphragmatic infarction. Potential exists for error, however. Suppose the diaphragmatic myocardial loss were sufficient to reduce R-wave amplitude but not to generate a Q wave. Thus, a diminutive R wave might be present, making the recognition of the diaphragmatic infarction very difficult (although S-T,T abnormalities may be helpful in suggesting that possibility). Such an inferior loss of myocardium may produce enough of a shift of axis to the left (headward) to meet the criterion for left-axis deviation. In this situation, infarction might generate QRS configuration in leads II, III, and aVF compatible with left anterior hemiblock. If precordial leads showed clockwise rotation (poor progression of R waves), the error would be assured; however, the configuration of S-T,T waves may provide the correct answer. In left anterior hemiblock, the inferior wall repolarizes "on time," while the anterior and lateral regions repolarize late. Thus, the T wave is upright in lead aVF in left anterior hemiblock. After diaphragmatic infarction, the T wave is most often inverted in that lead.

This patient, a 66-year-old woman, had suffered a diaphragmatic infarction. She developed unstable angina 9 years later and was admitted to the hospital. This EKG was therefore recorded 9 years after her infarction. Cardiac catheterization revealed total occlusion of the left anterior descending artery, 70% occlusion of the first diagonal branch of the left anterior descending artery, 50% occlusion of the circumflex artery, and 90% occlusion of the right coronary artery. A ventriculogram revealed modest global hypokinesia. Remarkably, the inferior and posterior walls of the left ventricle showed normal wall motion.

3. How can the EKG reveal a diaphragmatic infarction and the ventriculogram show diaphragmatic wall motion to be apparently normal?

ANSWER: Usually, Q-wave development implies depopulation of a wall sufficient to interfere with normal contractile behavior. It is possible, however, and apparently occurred in this instance, for the depopulation to be sufficiently severe to generate a loss of R waves and development of pathologic Q wave without sufficient damage to produce hypokinesis. It should be remembered that the infarction occurred 9 years prior to this study and that hypertrophy of the residual surviving myocardial cells in the diaphragmatic area may well have been sufficient to restore the appearance of normal wall motion.

The diminutive R wave seen in leads V_1 through V_5 can be attributed to the myocardial damage induced by obstruction of the left anterior descending artery and partial obstruction of its diagonal branch.

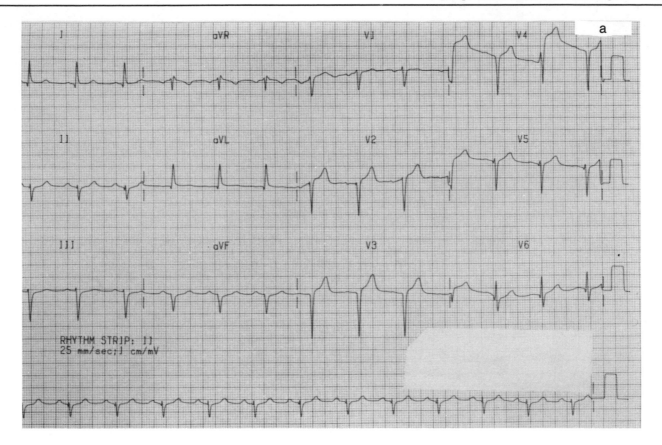

EKG 80

This patient, a 58-year-old man, developed severe pain in the anterior chest and left arm 30 min before admission to the emergency room where the first EKG was recorded. He had no past history of heart disease.

1. The first EKG (80a) is compatible with an anterior infarction. How old is the lesion?

ANSWER: Without old records for comparison, pathologic Q, QR, or QS configurations provide no temporal information; they might equally well represent fresh or old loss of cells. S-T,T configurations, on the other hand, are likely to be helpful in estimating the age of the process.

2. What do the S-T,T waves in record 80a indicate?

ANSWER: The rather tall T waves in leads V_2 through V_6 and the slight S-T elevation in leads V_2, V_3, and V_4 are far from diagnostic of an acute process, but they are sufficiently prominent to justify further tracings because the T waves could be minor variants of the "hyperacute T" phenomenon. The S-T elevations are within the extreme limits of normal variation: they do not exceed 2 mm elevation and they are concave-up.

3. Records 80b, c, and d confirm the presence of an acute infarction. Done on successive days, they present rapidly changing T-wave inversions. What is the meaning of the rapid deepening of the T waves?

ANSWER: This configuration indicates (1) progressive loss of cell population in the matrix of the acute infarction, with increasing repolarizing dipole deficiency; or (2) progressive alterations in the action potentials of surviving, but damaged, cells.

4. The restoration of upright T waves on the fourth day after infarction was not anticipated (record 80e). The possibility that this represented recurrent "hyperacute T" phenomenon came to mind but was discounted because of the persistence of the upright T waves during the next 3 days. A convincing explanation cannot be given for this abrupt recovery of

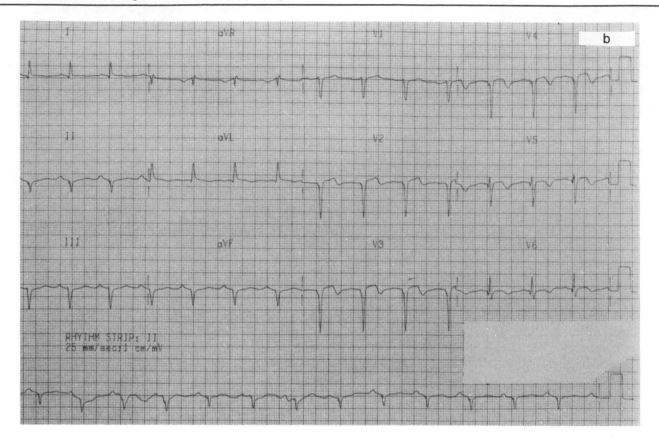

more normal T-wave configuration. Cardiac catheterization was performed on the day of the first record. What results would you expect?

ANSWER: One would expect high-grade obstruction of the left anterior descending artery. In view of the QS configuration in lead aVF, significant disease in the right or posterior descending artery would be a reasonable presumption. The widespread distribution of the abnormalities into the anterolateral region suggests circumflex or marginal disease. Indeed, both of these were found. The ventriculogram revealed marked hypokinesis of the apical, anterolateral, and inferior walls and of the adjoining regions. The surprising T-wave changes on the fourth, fifth, and sixth days, therefore, may have been reciprocal manifestations of posterior damage.

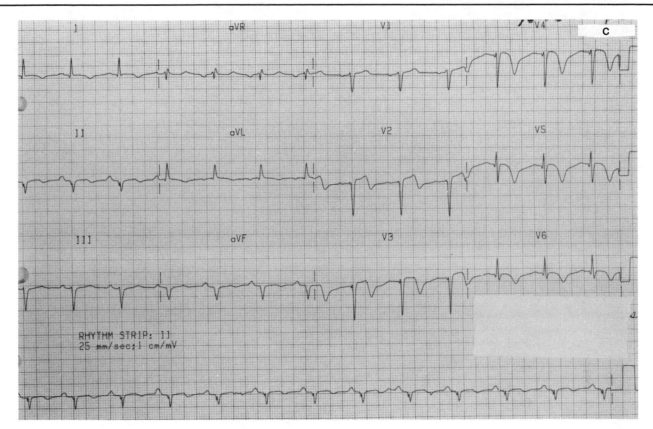

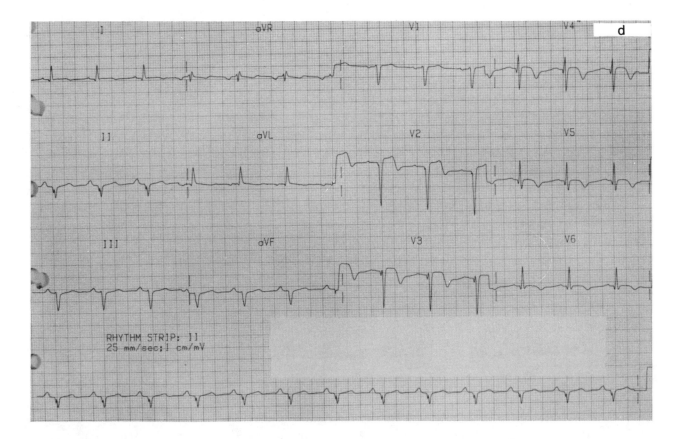

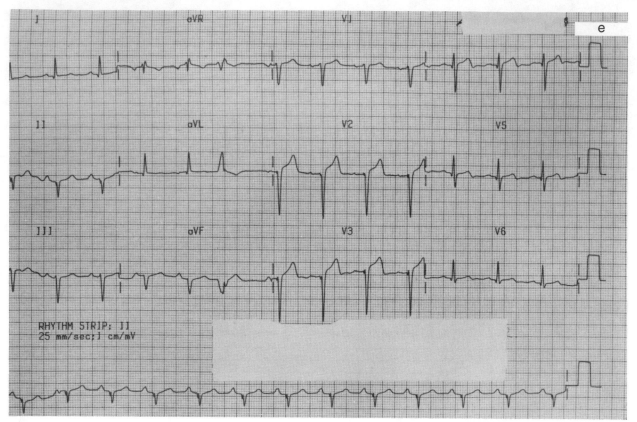

RHYTHM STRIP: II
25 mm/sec; 1 cm/mV

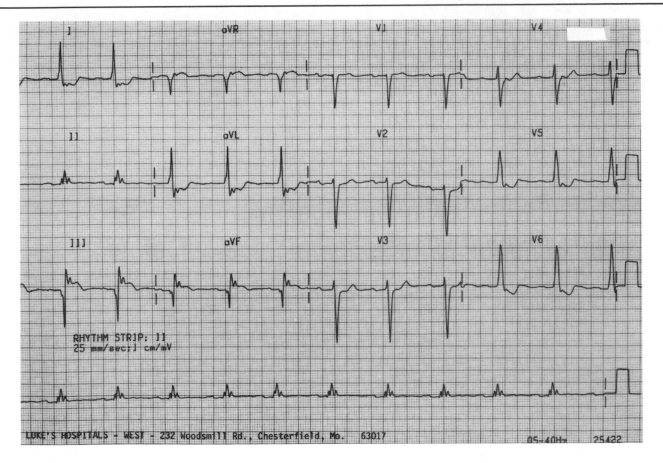

EKG 81

Note the QR-R' in leads III and aVF.

1. How would you visualize the state of the diaphragmatic myocardium?

ANSWER: The infarct is an interwoven complex of necrotic or fibrotic tissue, among which exists a population of surviving cells. The depolarization process advances through and around this area as through a maze. The peri-infarction block accounts for the significant intraventricular conduction delay (.20 sec).

2. What other information does this record provide?

ANSWER: The full-length-horizontal S-T deviations indicate 3 possibilities: (1) The infarction is acute, with a diastolic dipole generated by the presence of a diaphragmatic colony of injured cells with subnormal resting potential; (2) the infarction is old and aneurysmal, in which case the S-T deviation is a result of either stretching and thinning of the surviving intra-infarction sarcolemma or persistent ischemia with subnormal sarcolemmal produc-

tion of resting potential; or (3) there is an old infarction with a fresh injury overlying it.

One of the frequent complications of ventricular aneurysms is the occurrence of ventricular arrhythmias. At least two mechanisms are brought to mind by this record:

(1) The circuitous maze of conduction around and through this infarct would set the stage for a small re-entry circuit (page 53).

(2) The subnormal resting potentials of the stretched or ischemic cells are abnormally near threshold. These cells would not only be predisposed to ectopic beat generation, but would conduct slowly and further facilitate a slowly advancing re-entry circuit.

Finally, this record with tall R waves in leads I and aVL is compatible with left ventricular hypertrophy. Again we see a factor predisposing to arrhythmias: the larger the mass of the myocardium, the greater is the potential circuit for macro-reentry phenomenon.

The patient was admitted to the hospital with

unstable angina. Serial enzymes tests did not detect evidence of fresh infarction. She continued to have severe substernal pain requiring opiates and intravenous nitroglycerin for control. Cardiac catheterization revealed (1) left ventricular dilatation, (2) marked inferior and apical hypokinesis, (3) 90% obstruction of the right, 60% obstruction of the left main, and 100% obstruction of the left anterior descending coronary arteries. The persistent S-T deviations in this instance may represent aneurysmal deformity of the old infarction, although an aneurysm was not confirmed by ventriculography, or may represent the combination of old infarction plus fresh myocardial ischemic injury.

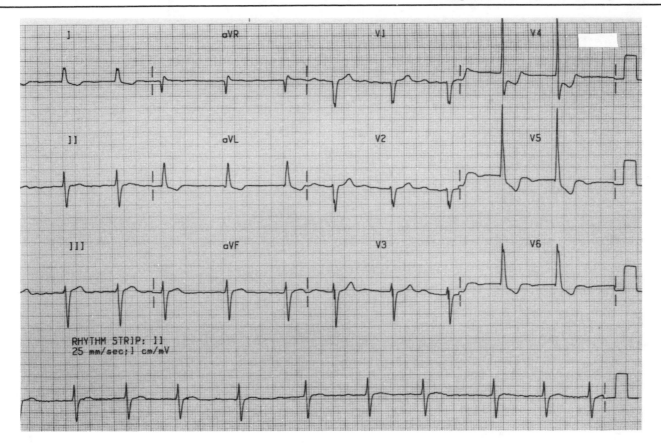

RHYTHM STRIP: II
25 mm/sec; 1 cm/mV

EKG 82

Left ventricular enlargement, left-axis deviation, and atrial fibrillation are readily apparent in this record.

1. What is the meaning of the 3-mm J point depression and down-sloping S-T segment in lead V_4?

ANSWER: In part, at least, this *full-length* S-T depression may result from conduction delay through the massive left ventricle. When phase 2 of the action potential has a down-slope, a difference in potential exists between the cells that depolarize early and those that follow (pages 76 and 100).

When full-length S-T depression occurs *without* intraventricular conduction delay in the presence of left ventricular hypertrophy, an ischemic mechanism must be considered, because the potential for cellular ischemia is inherent in ventricular hypertrophy (Case 40, page 128). Even if coronary capillaries multiply in the presence of hypertrophy, the spatial effects may engender cytoplasmic ischemia.

The subendocardial myocardium, most distal

from its blood supply, could reasonably be expected to be the most vulnerable and produce the S-T depression noted here.

Records of this type (EKG 82) require consideration of possible *acute* injury and justify comparison with serial records and older tracings.

2. What accounts for the left-axis deviation here? The question is raised to emphasize a point.

ANSWER: Small R waves appear in leads V_1, V_2, and V_3, but an abrupt increase in R-wave amplitude occurs in lead V_4. This, we believe, rules out the possibility of left anterior hemiblock where the circumferential and apex-to-base depolarization of the left ventricle produces gradual R-wave development from leads V_1 through V_6 (see page 41). Here, the left-axis orientation is produced by the large array of dipoles depolarizing toward the left shoulder through the free wall of the left ventricle. Two points deserve comment: (1) Thickness of the left ventricular wall increases from apex to base. With left ventricular hypertrophy, the greatest phalanx of depolarizing dipoles is found, therefore, in the basal half of the ventricle. (2) Termination of the Purkinje net near the equator of the left ventricle results in an angular vector of depolarization from the "end of the line" to the base. Thus, the large later forces are oriented superiorly and leftward.

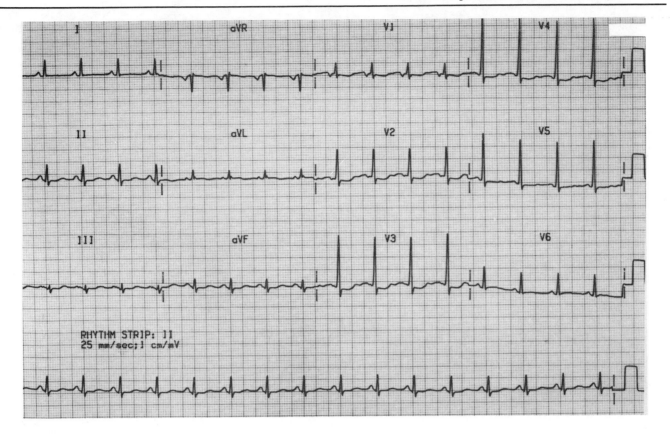

RHYTHM STRIP: II
25 mm/sec; 1 cm/mV

EKG 83

The depolarizing dipoles advancing toward leads V_1, V_2, and V_3 through the anterior septum and the adjacent anterior wall outnumber those advancing through the posterior septum and the adjoining posterior wall.

1. Why do we attribute the abnormal R waves to the septum and the nearby myocardium?

ANSWER: Because they occur within the first .02 to .04 sec.

2. Could this preponderance of anterior dipoles be the result of right ventricular enlargement?

ANSWER: Although the right ventricle might be better named the anterior ventricle, the prominent R waves in the precordial leads in the presence of right ventricular enlargement are most marked in lead V_1. Some have attributed this to extreme clockwise rotation secondary to expansion of the right ventricle with rotation of the left ventricle sufficient to direct some of its depolarizing dipoles toward lead V_1. Small R waves in lead V_2 are followed by progressively larger R waves in leads V_3 through V_6. The precordial leads in right ven-

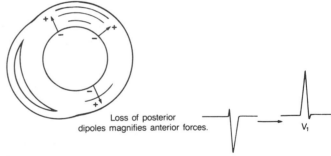

Loss of posterior dipoles magnifies anterior forces. V_1

Case 83

tricular hypertrophy therefore suggest erroneous electrode placement, with lead V_1 resembling normal lead V_6 and leads V_2 through V_6 each appearing shifted one position to the left (V_2 resembles normal V_1, V_3 resembles normal V_2, etc.).

Case 83 indicates a broad arc of excess anterior dipoles or deficient posterior dipoles and is therefore indicative of posterior infarction. The S-T depressions in leads V_2 through V_4 support this conclusion and suggest an active or an aneurysmal lesion.

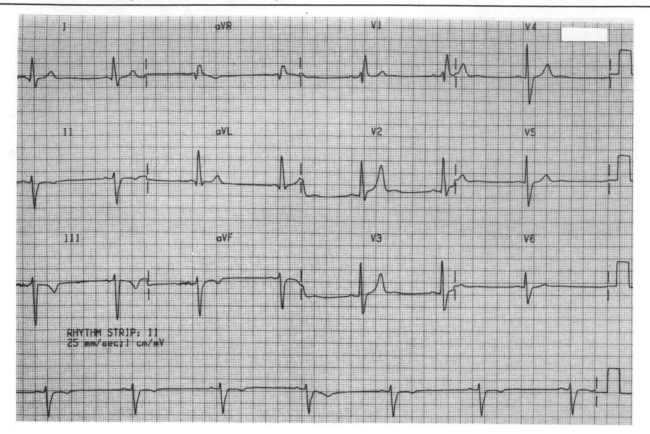

RHYTHM STRIP: II
25 mm/sec; 1 cm/mV

EKG 84

The combination of right bundle branch block and left anterior hemiblock is common. This record has been selected for discussion because of the tall T waves in leads V_2, V_3, and V_4.

1. Can they be attributed to the intraventricular conduction defects?

ANSWER: No. Almost without exception, leads overlying the area of conduction delay show inverted T waves because of the delay in re-polarization. *This* configuration indicates a loss of posterior-inferior repolarizing dipoles. Review of this patient's chart reveals that he had a well-documented diaphragmatic, anterolateral, and posterior infarction in 1970, accounting for the loss of the dipoles in this region. The loss of posterolateral dipoles has created an exaggeration of the now counterbalanced anteroseptal dipoles, with generation of tall T waves and R waves in leads V_1, V_2, and V_3.

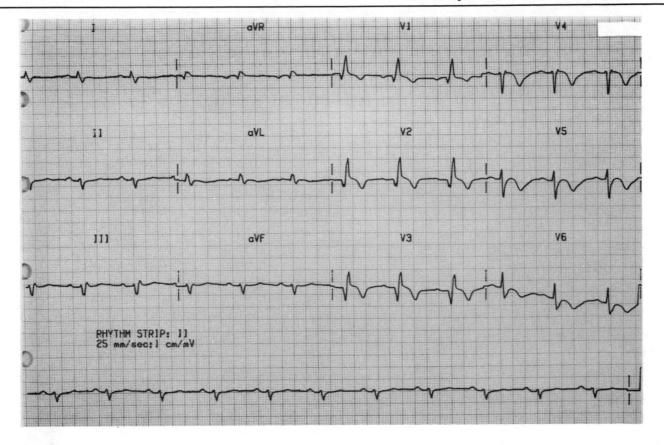

PHYTHM STRIP: II
25 mm/sec; 1 cm/mV

EKG 85

The peaks of prominent R waves in leads V_1, V_2, and V_3 in this record occur late (.09 to .10 sec) and follow .06-sec Q waves. Total QRS duration is .12 sec. The record reveals the common combination of right bundle branch block and left anterior hemiblock.

1. Why does no RsR' appear in leads V_1, V_2, and V_3?

ANSWER: The initial R wave in the RsR' of right bundle branch block is generated by anteroseptal depolarization. Its absence indicates septal infarction.

2. Note the upright T wave in leads II, III, and aVF. Is this to be expected in left anterior hemiblock?

ANSWER: Yes. Survival of the posterior hemibranch assures normal time of depolarization and repolarization of the inferior wall, activated by the posterior hemibranch. Sometimes, however, when complicated by right bundle branch block and the resultant delay in activation of the right ventricle, left anterior hemiblock is associated with inverted T waves in lead aVF. This phenomenon illustrates the potential overhang of the right ventricle over the inferior aspect of the heart.

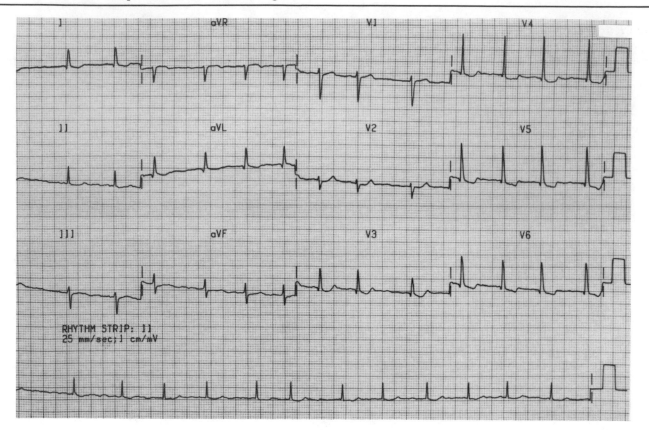

RHYTHM STRIP: II
25 mm/sec; 1 cm/mV

EKG 86

Electrocardiograms often present nonspecific as well as diagnostic abnormalities. It is important to make full use of all the findings and consider all the possibilities suggested. This record is a commonplace example.

1. What *diagnostic* abnormality is present?

ANSWER: Atrial fibrillation.

2. What *nonspecific* features are there?

ANSWER: The S-T,T abnormalities.

3. What do they suggest?

ANSWER: The *downsloping*, "almost *straight* enough to be along your ruler" configuration is seen most often in the presence of left ventricular "strain," which in turn, is the most frequent presentation of left ventricular enlargement. Digitalis produces similar downsloping, but *shortens* the S-T segment and Q-T interval because of its effects on the action potential (pages 65 and 66). Left ventricular hypertrophy or strain does not shorten the action potential or the Q-T interval. The Q-T interval shown here, .28 sec at a rate of 88 beats per minute, is shortened. The com-

bination of this form of S-T configuration and Q-T shortening is most suggestive of digitalis effect.

This type of S-T deviation seen with *normal* Q-T duration often indicates the presence of left ventricular strain hypertrophy (combined with) digitalis action, their Q-T effects cancelling each other.

Similar downsloping S-T and short Q-T configurations are produced by beta-adrenergic agents.

Atrial fibrillation brings to mind these possibilities: (a) atrial distension and increased left ventricular filling pressure resulting either from loss of inotropic function or from loss of compliance, (b) intrinsic atrial cellular damage, and (c) sinus nodal damage (in the wake of sickness of the sinus node, atrial fibrillation is analogous to a revolt among the troops when the captain has been killed).

This patient, a 76-year-old woman, was admitted to the hospital with atrial fibrillation of 3 weeks' duration and uncontrolled hypertension. On admission, her blood pressure was 215/115.

The medications being given to the patient at the time of this electrocardiogram included digoxin, .25 mg once a day. Digoxin blood concentration was 1.0 ng/ml. Thus, her electrocardiographic findings appeared to fit the clinical situation precisely in that she was a candidate for left ventricular strain and was receiving digitalis. The atrial fibrillation may have been the result of those factors suggested earlier in this discussion.

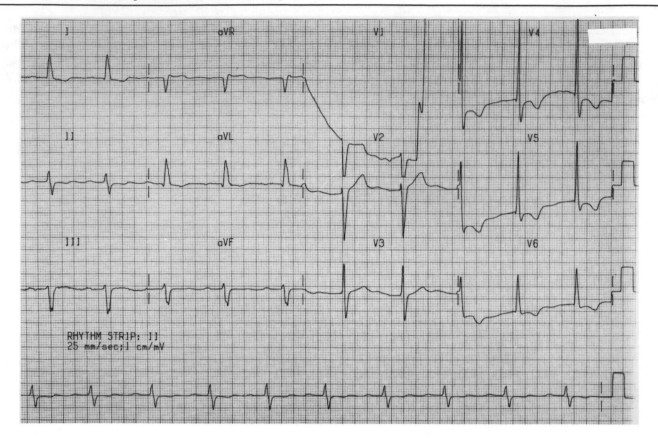

EKG 87

The QRS duration is .14 sec.

1. Does this record indicate left bundle branch block?

ANSWER: The Q wave in leads I, aVL, V_4, V_5, and V_6 assures left-to-right septal depolarization. That then excludes the diagnosis of left bundle branch block. The conduction delay here with increased voltage should be attributed instead to left ventricular hypertrophy. Had there been poor R-wave progression ("clockwise rotation"), the record, in addition, would have met the criteria for left anterior hemiblock.

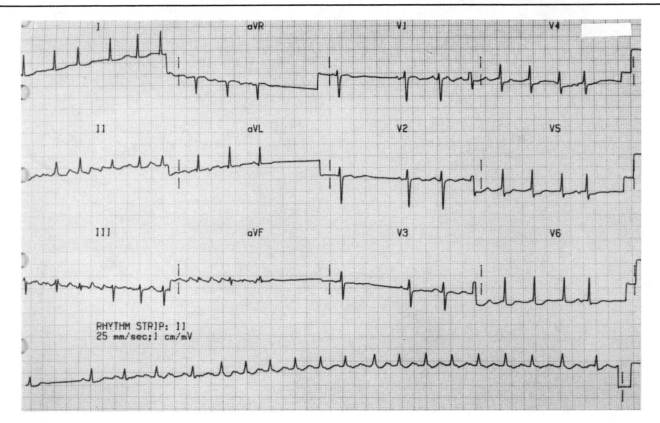

RHYTHM STRIP: II
25 mm/sec; 1 cm/mV

EKG 88

1. What are the atrial arrhythmias in this record?

ANSWER: The second beat in leads V_1 through V_3 is a sinus beat. It is followed by two ectopic beats. The first beat in leads V_1 through V_3 originates in another ectopic focus. In leads I, II, III, aVR, aVL, and aVF there is a brief run of flutter. In leads V_4, V_5 and V_6, the atrial pacemaker migrates once again. The rhythm strip (lead II) shows intermittent atrial tachycardia with predominant 2:1 A-V block.

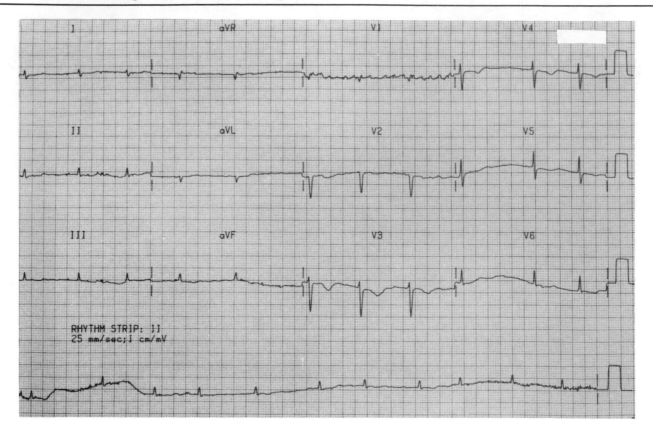

RHYTHM STRIP: II
25 mm/sec; 1 cm/mV

EKG 89

The abnormalities in this record suggest several possibilities.

1. What are the abnormalities?

ANSWER: (1) Atrial fibrillation. (2) Low voltage. (3) Clockwise rotation (or poor progression of R waves). (4) Inverted T waves in leads V_3 and V_4, and low T waves in all other leads.

2. What possibilities come to mind?

ANSWER: The focally inverted T waves suggest focal abnormality of repolarizing dipoles in the anteroseptal-anterior myocardium. Focal damage might be one of many types, but is most likely to be ischemic.

The low voltage also might reflect a variety of situations: obesity, pericardial effusion, myxedema, invasive myocardiopathy, but most frequently, chronic obstructive pulmonary disease.

The QR in lead V_1 is sufficient to be suggestive, but not diagnostic, of right ventricular enlargement.

The electrocardiographic abnormalities suggestive of right ventricular dilatation or en-largement include the following: (1) right-axis deviation and clockwise rotation (a nonspecific combination); (2) incomplete or complete right bundle branch block, which in fact, may be the result of elongation of the right ventricular free wall or dysfunction of the right bundle fibers; and (3) a striking presentation with a prominent R wave in lead V_1 followed by a configuration in leads V_2 and V_3 that resembles that seen in a normal V_1 and V_2; leads V_3 through V_6 reveal slowly progressive build-up of R waves with prominent S waves. The qR in lead V_1 may be so striking as to suggest a technical error, with V_6 recorded mistakenly as V_1 (page 197).

Atrial fibrillation may be the result of sick sinus state, atrial dilatation, or atrial myocardial damage.

Putting this all together, one might suspect chronic obstructive pulmonary disease with right ventricular enlargement. The patient's troubles might be compounded by coronary disease with anterior ischemic damage. In fact, this patient, a 90-year-old woman, suffered from pulmonary fibrosis and respiratory insufficiency. The results of echocardiographic examinations confirmed right ventricular and right atrial dilatation and tricuspid and pulmonic regurgitation. She died in respiratory failure. In view of her age, the possibility of an ischemic cause for the T-wave inversion in leads V_3 and V_4 is apparent.

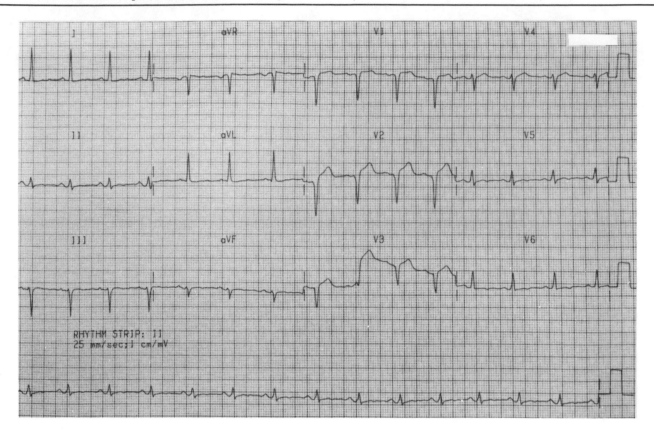

RHYTHM STRIP: II
25 mm/sec; 1 cm/mV

EKG 90

This patient was subjected to echocardiographic examination and to cardiac catheterization.

1. What findings would you predict from the EKG?

ANSWER: The echocardiogram should and did reveal apical and septal hypokinesis. The ventriculogram also demonstrated moderate hypokinesis of the anterolateral wall and septum. Obstruction of the left anterior descending system is predictable. Distal to the origin of the first diagonal artery was 100% obstruction of the left anterior descending coronary artery. There was 60% obstruction of its first diagonal branch.

2. Why were these areas of infarction hypokinetic rather than akinetic or dyskinetic?

ANSWER: This illustrates that infarction does not mean 100% loss of contractile cells in its matrix. The deeper the QS in leads V_1, V_2, and V_3 in this patient's EKG, the greater would be the depopulation in the infarct; but, once again, the appearance of QS does not mean total myocyte loss.

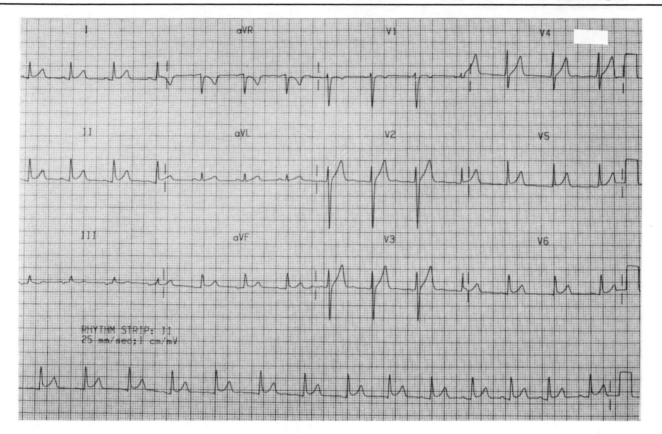

PHYTHM STRIP: II
25 mm/sec; 1 cm/mV

EKG 91

1. What does the S-T,T configuration suggest?

ANSWER: Probably a normal variant because (a) the S-T elevation is within normal limits, and (b) the T waves are normally upright.

2. Why "probably"?

ANSWER: Occasionally, the *early* stages of pericarditis may produce (a) slight S-T elevations in all leads except aVR, in which there may be a reciprocal S-T depression; and (b) normal T waves. Subsequent records in pericarditis would be expected to show T-wave inversions in multiple leads with upright T waves in lead aVR.

3. Why do these configurations occur in pericarditis?

ANSWER: Pericarditis is usually a widely distributed process, involving the epicardial surface of the ventricular "horseshoe." Lead aVR is likely to be the only lead oriented to face the endocardium and therefore presents S-T and T-wave changes that reciprocate the S-T,T abnormalities of the other 11 leads.

The P-R interval here is isoelectric.

4. Does this help distinguish the normal variant from epicarditis?

ANSWER: Yes. As noted elsewhere, the P-R segment is often depressed in pericarditis (11 leads other than aVR).

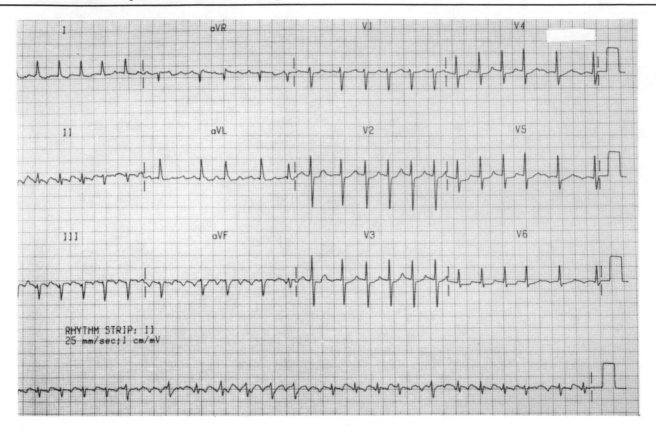

RHYTHM STRIP: II
25 mm/sec; 1 cm/mV

EKG 92

The atrial waves are seen best in leads II, III, aVL, and aVF. There is no isoelectric baseline between the atrial waves in these leads.

1. What mechanism might produce this configuration?

ANSWER: A macro-reentry or circus movement could generate this record.

2. Why are the atrial waves well formed in leads II, III, aVL, and aVF?

ANSWER: If the circus movement lies in a sagittal plane, the advancing positive pole and the retreating negative pole will "face" those leads with a longitudinal, anterior, and posterior component and will have their minimal projection on lateral leads.

3. Is this the common presentation of atrial flutter?

ANSWER: Yes. Flutter waves are often most clearly seen in inferior leads and in lead V_1.

4. What accounts for the less rapid and irregular ventricular rhythm?

ANSWER: Variable A-V block.

5. Why is this record classified as flutter and not as atrial tachycardia?

ANSWER: Arrhythmia is conventionally classified as atrial flutter when atrial rate is 250 to 350 beats per minute and no isoelectric baseline exists between beats (see pages 46 through 48).

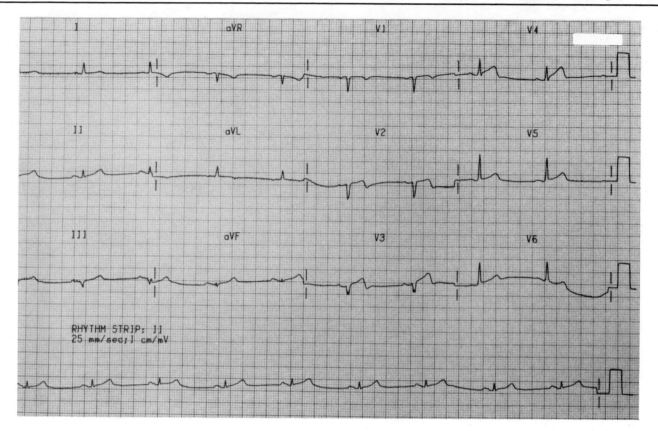

RHYTHM STRIP: II
25 mm/sec; 1 cm/mV

EKG 93

1. What would you do if your patient presented this record?

    ANSWER: (1) Compare it with earlier records to see whether the rS in leads V_2 and V_3 and the S-T and T configurations in leads V_2 through V_4 are new.

    (2) Relate it to clinical information.

2. Why?

    ANSWER: The S-T,T in leads V_2 through V_4 is compatible with an anteroseptal anterior ischemic process that may be of recent onset. This possibility would require that further records be made, unless older tracings and clinical data indicate an *old* lesion.

3. Do the minute r waves in leads V_2 and V_3 exclude the possibility of infarction?

ANSWER: Not at all. Necrotic loss of cells may be sufficiently severe to reduce the depolarizing mass and thus reduce the R wave, without being sufficiently massive to produce pathologic Q waves. *Thus, infarction without pathologic Q waves is a frequent phenomenon.*

4. What else may yield infarction without Q waves?

ANSWER: (a) Subendocardial infarction that lies within the self-cancelling inner zone (page 10); (b) infarction of opposing walls may reduce dipole populations equally, so that the deficit in neither wall is evident; and (c) patchy necrosis intermingled with hypertrophic cells may leave a normal residual dipole census in the region.

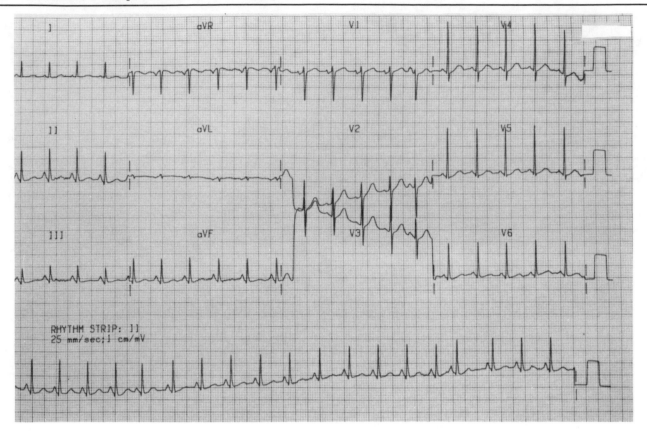

EKG 94

This record shows a P-R interval of .10 sec and peaked P waves in leads II, III, and aVF. The P waves suggest right atrial enlargement. Let your imagination run free and propose an explanation for the accelerated atrioventricular conduction.

ANSWER: The patient may have pulmonary disease and may be receiving a beta-adrenergic drug or theophylline. Both types of agents frequently shorten the P-R interval.

The patient did indeed have chronic obstructive pulmonary disease and intrinsic asthma. Medications being administered at the time the electrocardiogram was taken included prednisone, oral theophylline, intravenous theophylline, and metaproterenol.

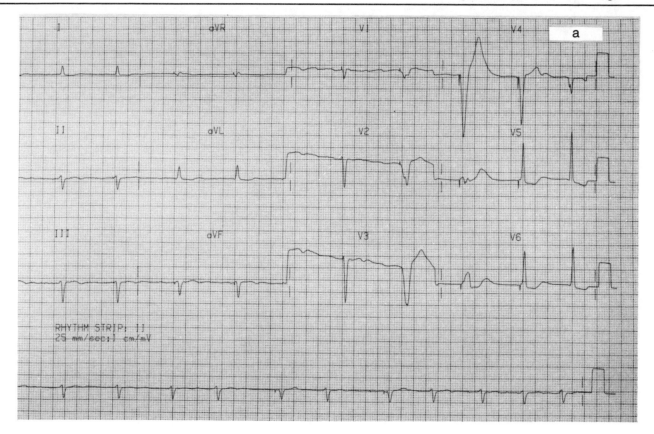

EKG 95a

1. Where is the pacemaker electrode situated?

ANSWER: The location of the electrode, like the "birthplace" of premature contractions, can be estimated by the QRS configuration in three leads, one longitudinal (aVF), one horizontal (V_5 or V_6), and one oriented in an anterior-posterior axis (V_1 or V_2). The lead in which a small initial R wave is followed by a large S wave overlies the electrode. The small initial R wave is generated in the ventricular wall adjacent to the electrode; the large, wide S wave is produced by the spread of depolarization from its point of origin. In this case, the electrode lies on the caudal wall of the ventricles, on the right, anteriorly. The electrode lies on the right of the septum (see Case 95a). Note the QS of pacemaker beat in lead V_2 and the rS of the intrinsic beat in lead V_2.

2. Why is there a virtually isoelectric period following the pacemaker blip in leads V_5 and V_6?

ANSWER: The net vector of early depolarization is directed at 90° to the axis of leads V_5 and V_6.

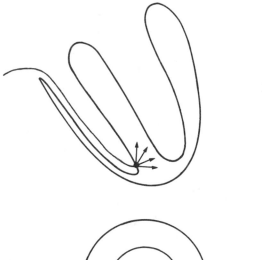

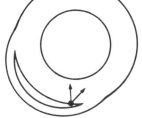

Case 95a

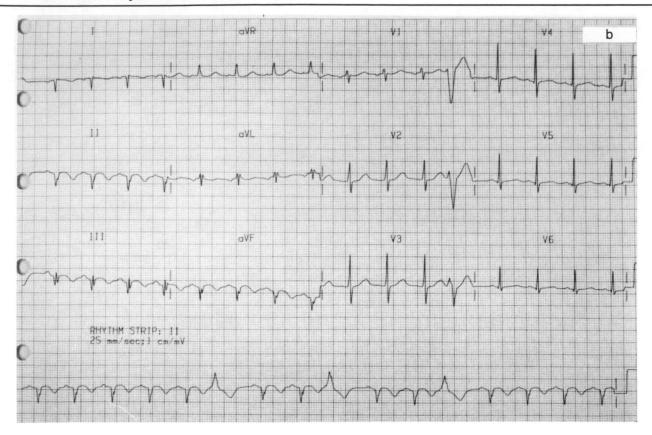

EKG 95b

In this record, premature ventricular contractions can be analyzed in the same way as were the pacemaker beats in EKG 95a.

1. How does the diaphragmatic posterior infarct influence the pacemaker QRS configuration? Particularly intriguing is the upright QRS configuration of premature ventricular contractions in lead II. How can the premature ventricular contraction produce an upright QRS complex in lead II when the sinus beat, as a result of the diaphragmatic posterior infarction, generates a QS in lead II?

ANSWER: The premature ventricular contractions in leads V_1 through V_3 indicate an anterior origin. The upright configuration of the premature ventricular contractions in lead II indicate a basal origin, with depolarization advancing toward the apex through the surviving ventricular myocardium.

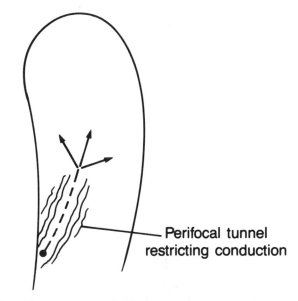

Perifocal tunnel restricting conduction

Case 95b

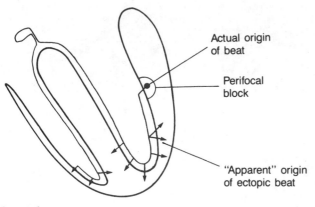

Actual origin
of beat

Perifocal
block

"Apparent" origin
of ectopic beat

Case 95b

2. Do these comments mean the electrocardi-
    ogram identifies with precision the focus from
    which ectopic beats arise?

ANSWER: Often, electrophysiologic studies pin-
point a "birthplace" of ectopy that is not the
site suggested by the electrocardiogram. It is
reasonable to suspect "tunneling" of the ectopic depolarization over fibers of the Purkinje
system or by way of "insulated" segments of
myocardium to remote areas from which the
depolarization bursts forth (Case 95b).

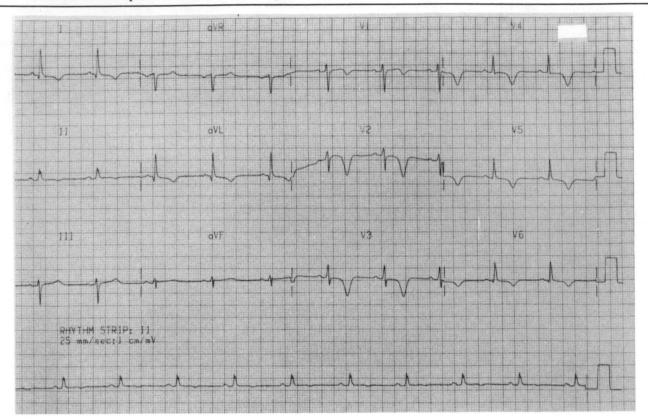

EKG 96

Symmetrically inverted T waves are often produced by an ischemic process.

1. What fundamental abnormality do they represent?

ANSWER: An abnormality in phase 3 of the action potential without an abnormality of resting potential or of phase 2 (because no S-T abnormality is present). Two possibilities exist here. The problem may be transmural, with delay or depletion of repolarizing dipoles from epicardium (first part of T wave) to endocardium. In this case, the anterior wall is generating fewer positive charges facing the electrode than the negative charges produced simultaneously by the posterior wall. The second possibility is that subendocardial cell damage accelerates repolarization of the inner myocardial layers, causing the repolarizing dipoles to present negative poles to the precordial electrodes.

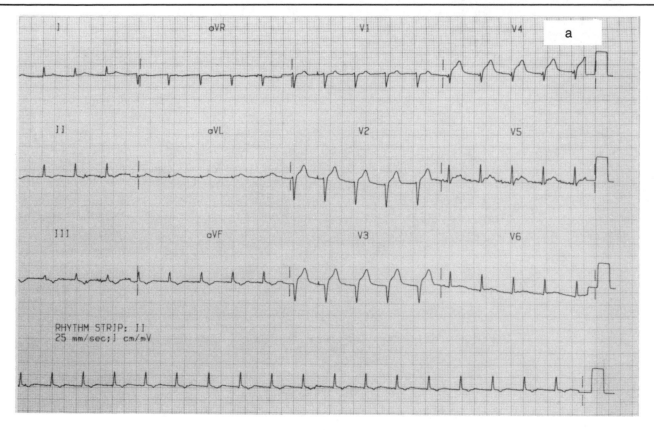

RHYTHM STRIP: II
25 mm/sec; 1 cm/mV

EKG 97

Records 97a and 97b are a continuation of a series of records of a patient whose earlier tracings were shown as EKG 77a and b. When comparing 97a with 77b recorded 2 days earlier, S-T,T changes have occurred.

1. Are they favorable?

ANSWER: The subsidence of the S-T depression in leads II, III, and aVF and the partial subsidence of the S-T elevation in leads V_1 through V_5 indicate a reduction in the intensity of the injury to surviving cells. (This colony of severely damaged cells is experiencing a recovery of either (a) a more normal resting potential, or (b) a more normal phase 2 of the action potential, as discussed previously.) A word might be said about the concave upward configuration of the S-T in leads V_2 through V_5 in 97a as compared with the configuration seen in 77b. As a general rule (and like all general rules, there are many exceptions), the more convex upward an elevated S-T segment, the more likely it is to reflect a pathologic process. The normal variant S-T elevation is typically concave upward, whereas the "bad"

news or injury-related S-T is more likely to be convex upward.

2. EKG 97a was recorded 1 day after 4-vessel coronary bypass operation. Record 97b was made 8 days later. What arrhythmia appeared in 97b? Are you surprised?

ANSWER: Atrial flutter appeared, which was not a great surprise. Atrial arrhythmias are commonplace in patients immediately after coronary bypass operation. In some patients, arrhythmias may reflect atrial dilatation resulting from ventricular dysfunction. In others, they may represent ischemic atrial damage; sympathomimetic excess, either spontaneous or drug related; or pericardial inflammation following surgical manipulation. Normally, the parietal pericardium is adherent to the atrial epicardium. Therefore, inflammation of the pericardium may involve the atrial myocardium and its latent pacemaker cells. This patient was receiving a sympathomimetic agent following an intrapericardial operation. Thus, several factors may have exerted cumulative effects on the atrial myocardium.

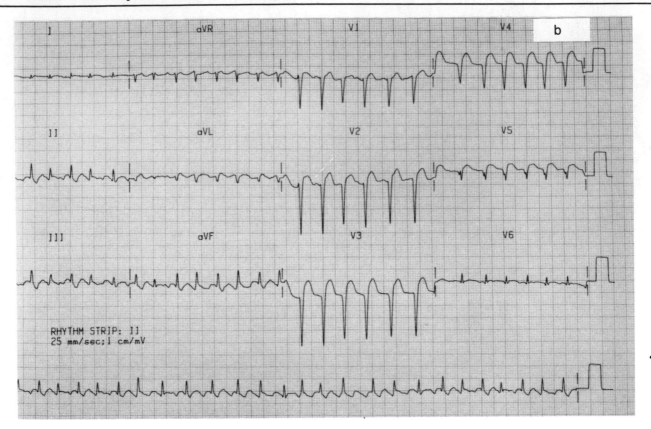

RHYTHM STRIP: II
25 mm/sec; 1 cm/mV

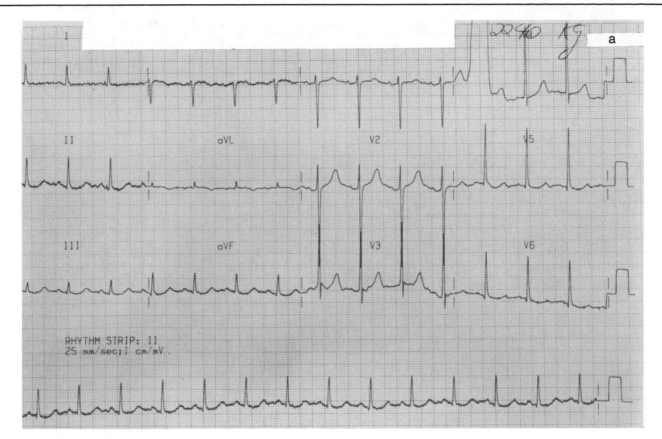

EKG 98

These records dated 7/15 (98a), 7/16 (98b), and 7/17 (98c) reveal interesting sequential changes, including intraventricular conduction delay and S-T,T alterations, on the last one (dated 7/17).

1. What chemical analysis would you order on receiving the record of 7/17?

ANSWER: You would be well advised to order a determination of serum potassium level. This patient was in a state of severe renal failure, with creatinine level at 6.8 mEq/L. On 7/15, his potassium was 3.6 but on 7/17 rose to 6.3 mEq/L. The changes noted on that date are seen frequently in the presence of hyperkalemia: notably, the widening of the QRS complex as a result of hyperkalemic intraventricular conduction delay and the peaked T waves because of steepening of the downslope of phase 3 of the action potentials (page 55). The striking depression of the S-T segments in leads V_4, V_5, and V_6 in 98c is worthy of emphasis, however. One can account for this S-T depression by recalling that phases 2 and 3 of the action potential are tipped down sharply in the presence of hyperkalemia; therefore, in the presence of the intraventricular conduction delay, relation to the first-to-last cells' action potentials resembles that seen in other intraventricular conduction disorders. As noted earlier, in the presence of left bundle branch block, for example, a downsloping phase 2 is responsible for a depression of the S-T segment from the J point to its termination. If phase 2 is horizontal while phase 3 descends steeply in hyperkalemia, the delay in conduction from the first-to-the-last cell will not disturb the isoelectric S-T segment while significantly disturbing phase 3 and the T wave (see page 100).

Note the absence of a recognizable P wave on record 98c. Hyperkalemia has been found to cause sinoatrial block with loss of the P wave but with preservation of conduction of depolarization from the S-A node to the A-V node over the internodal pathways. Thus, this patient, with a rate of 110 beats per minute, can be expected to have a sinus nodal pacemaker despite the fact that no P waves are seen.

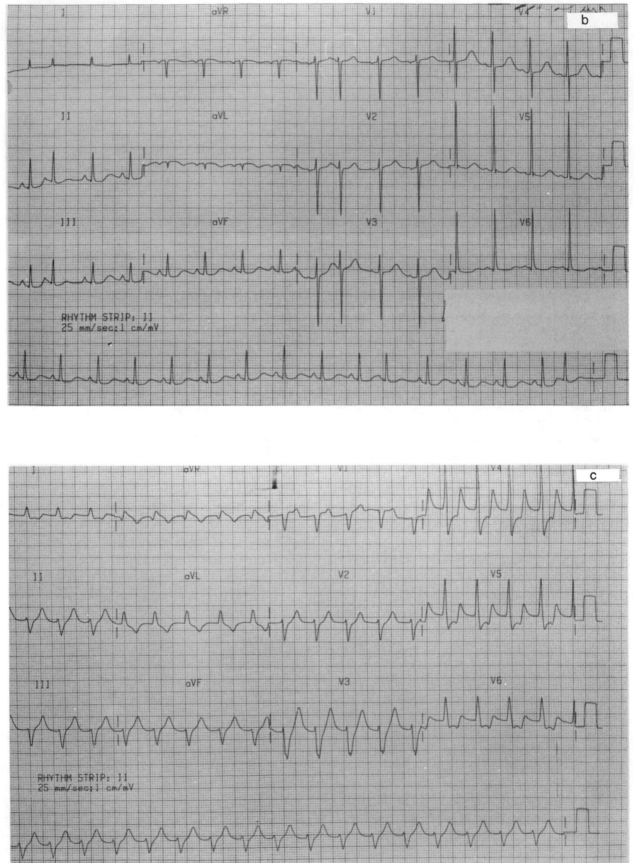

RHYTHM STRIP: II
25 mm/sec; 1 cm/mV

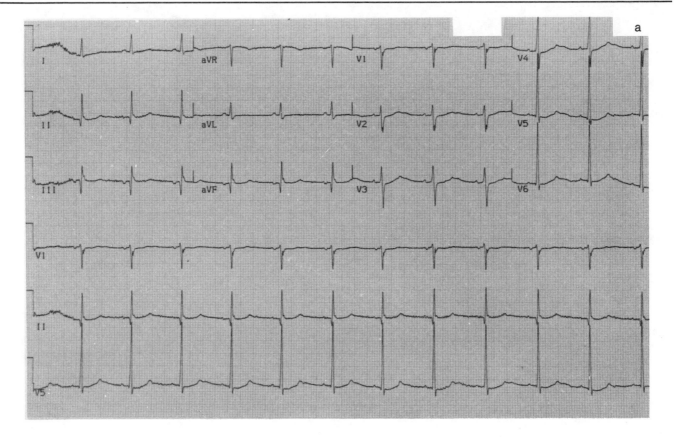

EKG 99

This patient, a 61-year-old man, had an acute myocardial infarction 7 years prior to the recording of these electrocardiograms. Following the infarction, he had been subjected to 3-vessel coronary bypass operation. He continued to have intermittent chest pain. Three weeks prior to these recordings, total hip repair had been performed. His postoperative course was complicated by recurrent fever with suspected left lower lobe pneumonitis. The results of pulmonary angiogram had shown no evidence of pulmonary embolism. Arterial oxygen pressure had been 50 mm Hg. The first record (99a) showed abnormalities compatible with an old diaphragmatic myocardial infarction.

1. How would you analyze the S-T changes seen on the second record (99b)?

ANSWER: In this patient with known coronary disease, these abnormalities were compatible with acute coronary insufficiency. The region involved would lie in the anterior subendocardial zone or in the posterior myocardium (pages 28 to 35).

2. In view of the aforementioned clinical information, what additional possibilities come to mind?

ANSWER: Although this record indicates localized myocardial injury and the problem may be acute impairment of flow through the left anterior descending or posterior descending coronary arteries, the problem also may have resulted from systemic hypoxia superimposed on a stable, albeit subnormal, coronary flow through either of these vessels. It is helpful to remember that S-T deviations of this sort are the electrocardiographic corollaries of myocardial *cyanosis* or *pallor*.

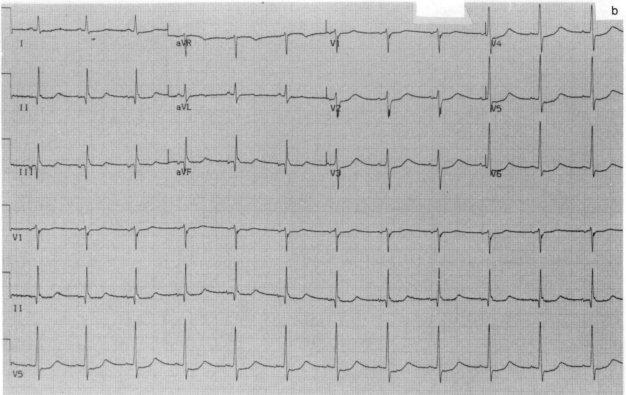

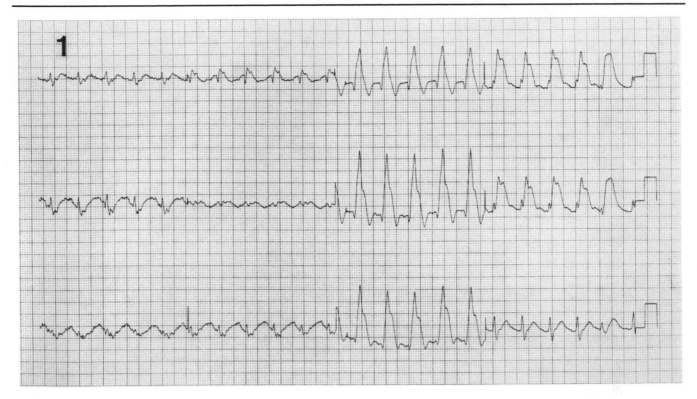

EKG 100

This patient was admitted with an acute my-ocardial infarction complicated by right bundle branch block. EKG 100a was recorded in the emer-

gency room. EKG 100b was recorded 2 days later in the intensive care unit. EKG 100c was recorded 5 days after record b and EKG 100d was recorded 3 days later. This series of records presents typical

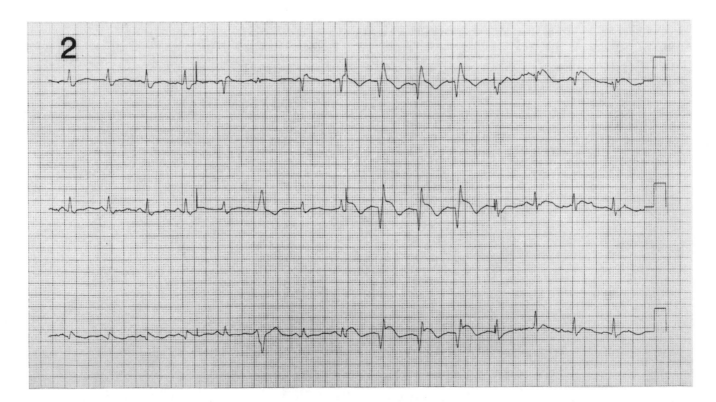

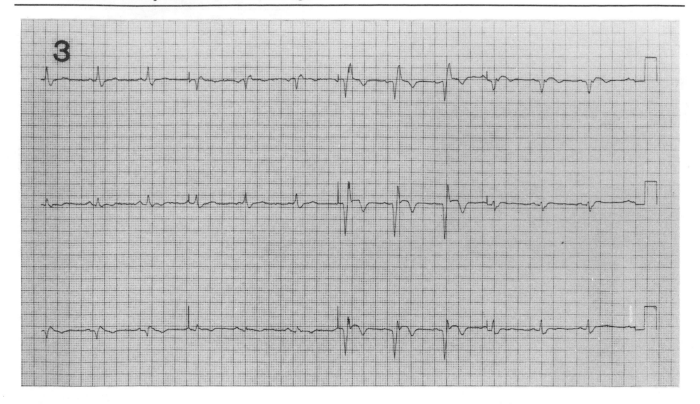

changes in the evolution of an acute myocardial infarction. Direct your attention to the sequential changes in the S-T segments and the T waves.

1. Do the increasingly abnormal T waves seen in leads V_2 through V_5 suggest that this patient has had further damage after admission to the hospital?

ANSWER: No. This record does not indicate further damage despite the fact that the T waves become increasingly abnormal. As shown in

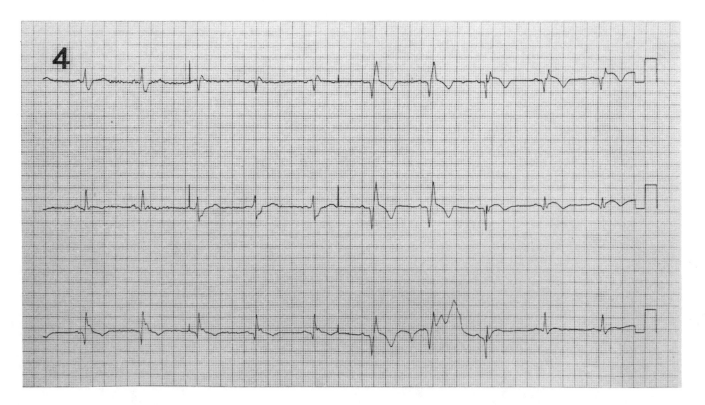

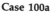

+ Normal resting potential and positive surface charge.

+ Injured cells with diminished resting potential and surface charge.

● Dead cells

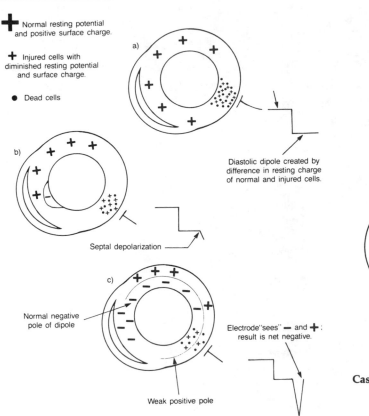

a)

Diastolic dipole created by difference in resting charge of normal and injured cells.

b)

Septal depolarization

c)

Normal negative pole of dipole

Electrode "sees" **—** and **+** : result is net negative.

Weak positive pole

Case 100a

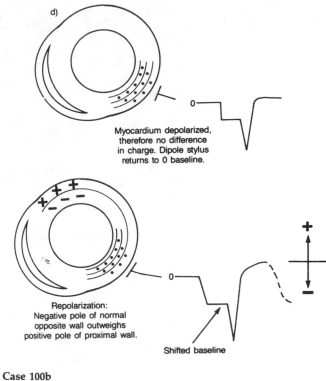

d)

Myocardium depolarized, therefore no difference in charge. Dipole stylus returns to 0 baseline.

Repolarization: Negative pole of normal opposite wall outweighs positive pole of proximal wall.

Shifted baseline

Case 100b

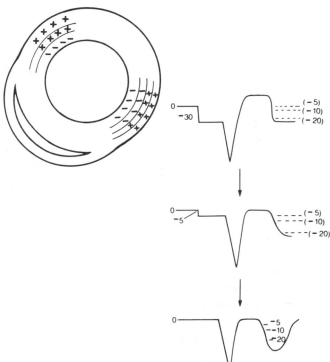

Case 100c

Case 100a and b, the true zero baseline in each of these records is probably at the level of the S-T segments, and the T wave in relation to that true baseline has not shown progressive inversion. The return of the S-T segments to normal implies disappearance of a population of severely damaged cells with subnormal resting potential. As that population of cells either recovered or died, the diastolic dipole generated between injured cells with subnormal resting potential and normal cells with normal resting potential disappears. With its disappearance, diastolic baseline returns to normal and the illusion of S-T elevation disappears. As the true zero S-T segment returns to the level of the diastolic baseline, the T wave appears to become more deeply inverted, whereas in fact, it has not changed in its relation to the true baseline (Case 100c).

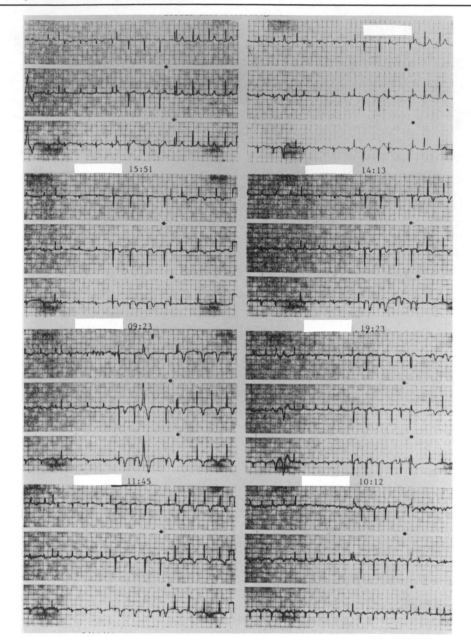

EKG 101

This panel of serial tracings reveals apparent loss of anteroseptal, anterior myocardial cells. The process appears active.

1. To what would you ascribe the abnormalities?

ANSWER: This appears to be the classic presentation of an acute myocardial infarction. This patient was studied carefully and found to have focal wall-motion abnormalities compatible with an anteroseptal lesion. CK-MB concentrations remained normal, however, and technetium pyrophosphate scan revealed no sign of infarction. Postmortem examination revealed regional eosinophilic myocarditis.

This case was chosen for discussion because it serves to emphasize two points: (a) an inflammatory process can so disorder sarcolemmal function as to mimic an infarction; (b) myocarditis may be segmental or regional, rather than global. Typically, myocarditis produces nonspecific T-wave abnormalities. Their presence is most helpful in the recognition of the nature of the process when they are found in many leads, suggesting a widespread or global process.

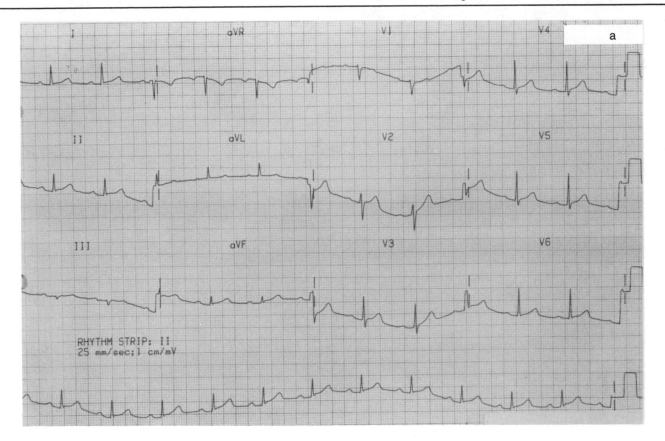

RHYTHM STRIP: II
25 mm/sec; 1 cm/mV

EKG 102

1. What are the notable features of this series (a to f)?

ANSWER: In records 102a and b, the S-T segments are very slightly elevated in all leads except V_1 and aVR. The elevation is within the limits of normal variation and the T waves are also within normal limits. Therefore, these first two records might be considered normal variants. It should be emphasized, however, that the constellation of S-T elevation in all leads facing the epicardium and S-T depression in the only lead facing into the ventricular endocardium is characteristic of pericarditis. When the configuration found in the first two records is seen, one should consider additional serial records to seek evidence of such a process. In the present case, a pericardial friction rub and echocardiographic demonstration of fluid within the pericardial space were asso-ciated with S-T,T changes compatible with an active epicardial process. The global distribution of the process is significant.

2. Could one distinguish between pericarditis and myocarditis here?

ANSWER: No. Because the S-T,T changes of pericarditis are the result of subepicardial myocarditis.

3. Could one distinguish between an ischemic process and an inflammatory one?

ANSWER: In truth, one could not distinguish between a widespread ischemic and a widespread inflammatory process. The almost global distribution of the S-T,T abnormalities, however, would favor a diagnosis of pericardial and myocardial inflammation. Neither the pericardial friction rub nor the pericardial effusion would *exclude* an ischemic process as the cause.

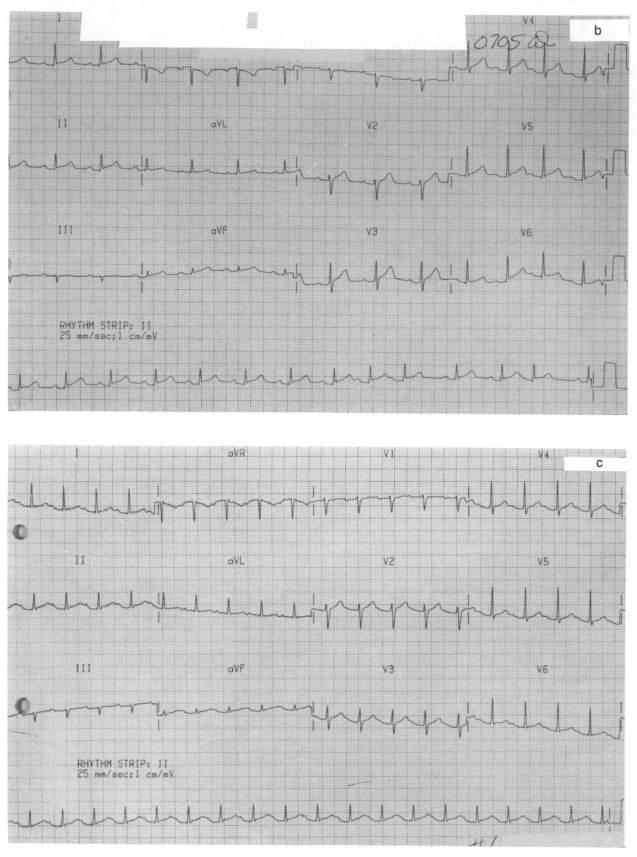

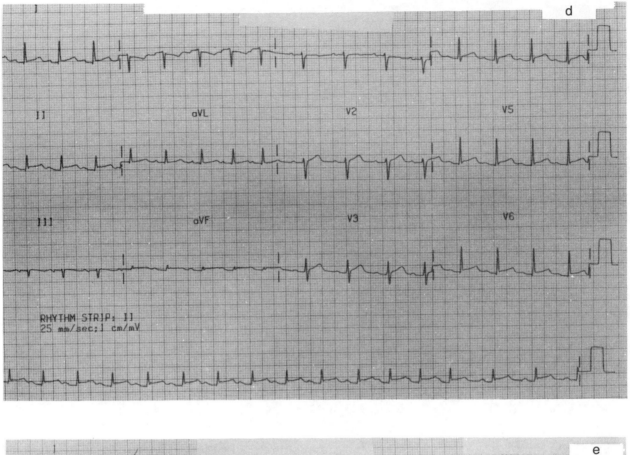

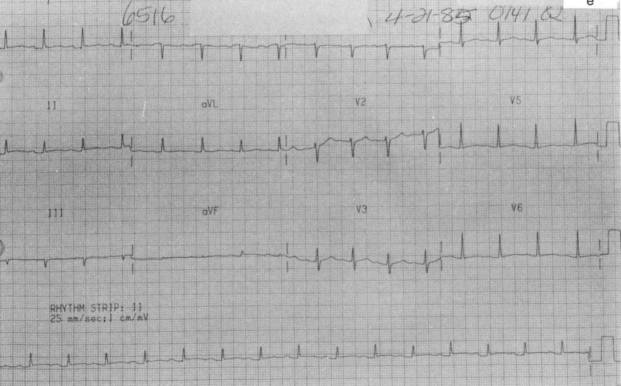

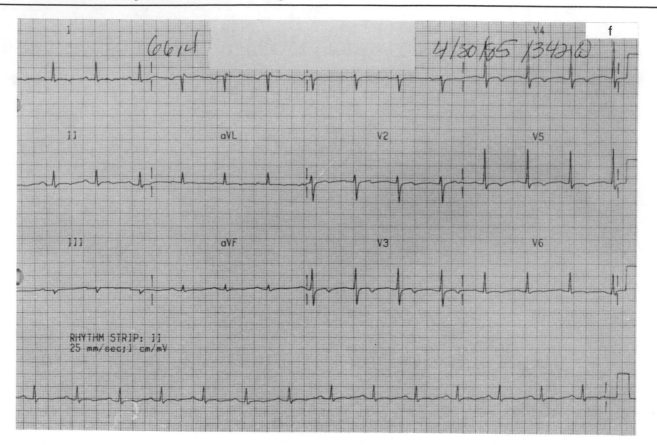

RHYTHM STRIP: II
25 mm/sec; 1 cm/mV

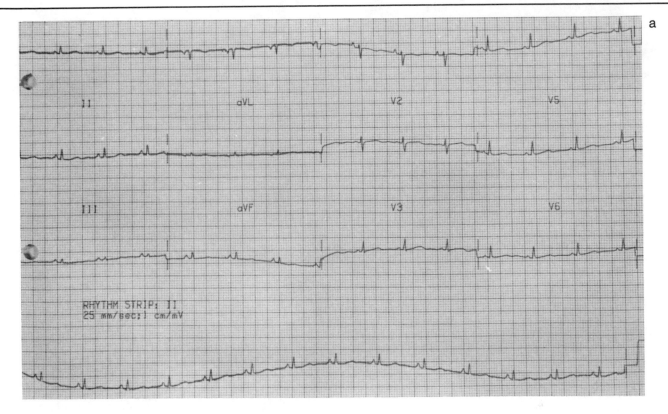

a

RHYTHM STRIP: II
25 mm/sec: 1 cm/mV

EKG 103

Voltage in record 103a is low (less than 5 mm positive or negative deflection of QRS in leads I, II, and III). The S-T,T configuration is normal.

1. What may have produced this abnormality without S-T,T change?

ANSWER: The common possibilities include (a) hyper-inflated lungs, (b) obesity, and (c) pericardial effusion.

The second EKG (103b) was recorded 6 days after the first. A large volume of pericardial fluid was removed in the interval between records. Note the P waves in each record.

2. What do they suggest?

ANSWER: Right atrial enlargement. This patient was afflicted with chronic obstructive pul-

monary disease of sufficient severity to produce recognizable right atrial enlargement (but it was not responsible for the low voltage).

Unlike the records of the preceding patient with pericarditis, the tracings of this patient with pericardial effusion revealed no S-T,T abnormality.

3. How can this be?

ANSWER: Pericardial effusion, without associated myocardial inflammation or damage does not affect the electrical behavior of myocardial cells and, therefore, does not disturb the S-T,T generation. It can be expected, therefore, to be manifested only by a reduction in voltage, as seen in this instance.

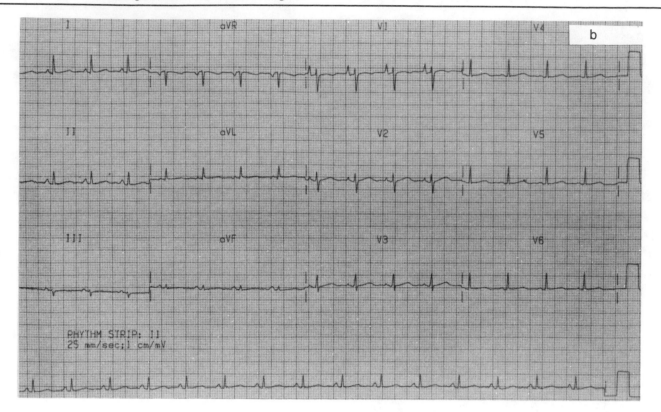

PHYTHM STRIP: II
25 mm/sec;1 cm/mV

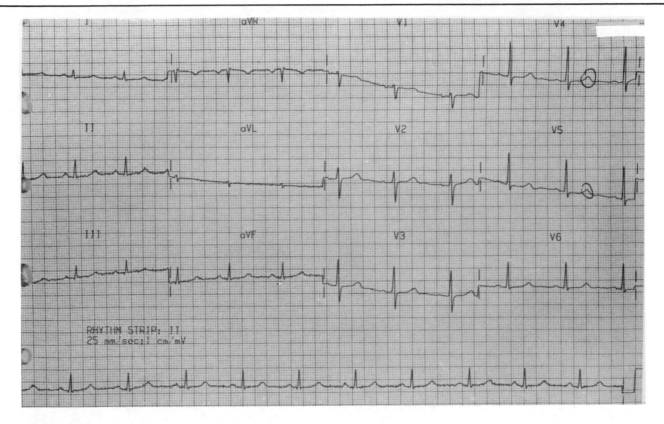

EKG 104

The electrocardiogram may serve as an indicator, or raise suspicions, of several metabolic abnormalities. The Q-T interval in this record is prolonged, .46 sec at a rate of 64 beats per minute.

1. Because the QRS duration is normal, .08 sec, what must the Q-T extension represent?

ANSWER: Action potential prolongation.

Because the durations of the QRS complex and the T wave are normal and they are the products of phases 1 and 2 (QRS) and 3 (T wave), the prolongation can be attributed to lengthening of phase 2 (S-T segment).

2. What ion bears a close relation to phase 2?

ANSWER: Calcium. Hypocalcemia may be reflected in S-T and Q-T prolongation. In this case, hypocalcemia was documented, with ionized calcium concentration at 4.29 (normal limits are 4.60 to 5.30).

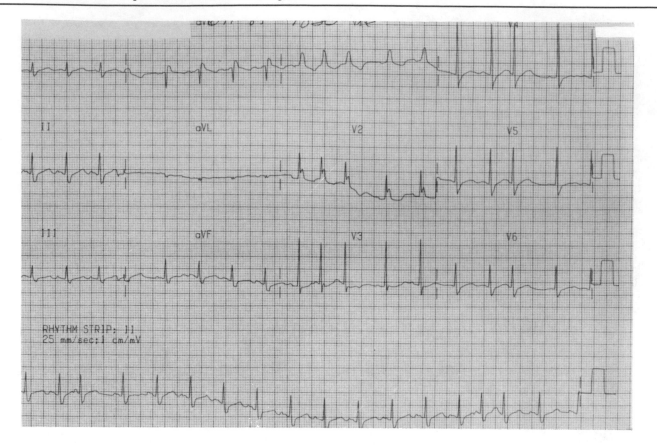

EKG 105

This record presents a subtle hint worthy of note. Despite bundle branch block with QRS duration of .12 sec, the Q-T interval is not prolonged; indeed, it is .36 sec, within normal limits for the heart rate.

1. What might act to shorten the Q-T interval?
ANSWER: Many influences, including (a) sympathomimetic stimulation, (b) digitalis, and (c) hypercalcemia.

In this instance, hypercalcemia (11.2 to 12.7 mg/dl) was present. No digitalis was present in blood analyses.

Because hypocalcemia lengthens phase 2 and the S-T segment, that phase 2 and S-T segment are shortened by hypercalcemia is no surprise. In this case, the "full-blown" picture of hypercalcemia with downsloping, very short S-T segment was not seen. That configuration resembles the S-T,T change induced by digitalis action, but the S-T shortening produced by hypercalcemia may be much greater than that generated by digitalis.

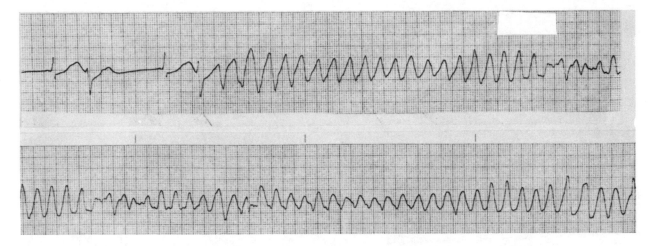

EKG 106

1. This monitor strip was recorded in this presence of which of the following drugs?
    (a) Digitalis
    (b) Quinidine
    (c) Furosemide
    (d) Lidocaine

ANSWER: This curious multiform ventricular tachyarrhythmia is an example of torsade de pointes—so named because one observer believed the varying QRS complexes were best described as a "turning of the points." This phenomenon occurs most often in the presence of Q-T prolongation. It is not surprising, therefore, to find it an occasional complication in patients receiving those drugs which lengthen the Q-T interval, most commonly quinidine and other Type IA drugs. This patient was subjected to electrophysiologic studies, and Wolff-Parkinson-White syndrome was identified. When quinidine was discontinued, torsade did not recur.

Curiously, this phenomenon occurs most often with low-dose rather than with "toxic" levels of these agents and especially in the presence of hypokalemia.

2. What could be the mechanism of the slowly changing configuration in this unique form of ventricular tachycardia?

ANSWER: Many have speculated on this question. A possible mechanism takes into account its occurrence when one or more factors prolong the Q-T interval. Figure I-123 indicates the birth of a premature ventricular contraction, with expansion of the depolarization into the adjacent myocardium in a sunburst fashion.

If the Q-T interval were unequally prolonged around the perimeter of the place of origin of the premature ventricular contraction, the second beat of a run of premature depolarizations would proceed in some directions and not in others (see Figs. I-127 and I-131). If this phenomenon occurred progressively, there would be a gradual "rotation" or "turning" of the direction of depolarization, and records such as this patient's would result.

Another possibility exists. If the subendocardial myocardial Q-T interval and refractory period progressively increased during a "run" of tachycardia, the ectopic depolarization might be conducted retrograde over the Purkinje net and appear to originate in a progressive migratory fashion (see Fig. I-124).

3. Why should "progressive" refractoriness and Q-T prolongation occur?

ANSWER: The answer may lie in the tachycardia itself. Tachycardia may, itself, induce refractoriness and block. Why the area of refractoriness might expand unevenly is intriguing. One might propose an uneven distribution of Q-T interval in the first place. Thus areas A, B, C, for instance, might conduct an ectopic depolarization from its origin. With rapid firing, A might be refractory to beat 2, and then area B might be refractory to beat 3. Thus, a varying exit block would account for the multiform ventricular tachycardia.

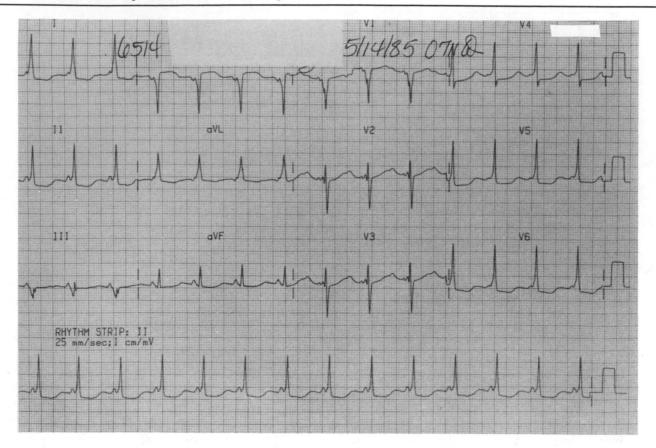

EKG 107

This is another electrocardiogram from the preceding patient with torsades de pointes. There are indications of Wolff-Parkinson-White syndrome.

1. What are they?

ANSWER: (a) delta waves.

   (b) short P-R interval.

   (c) prolonged QRS complex.

   (d) nonspecific S-T,T configuration.

2. Where would you expect the pre-excitation bridge to be located?

ANSWER: Studies in this patient confirmed a Kent bundle located in the anteroseptal region. The negative delta wave in lead III and the positive delta waves in leads V_4 through V_6 are evidence of the superior leftward direction of the pre-excitation wave, presumably initiated on the right side of the interventricular septum.

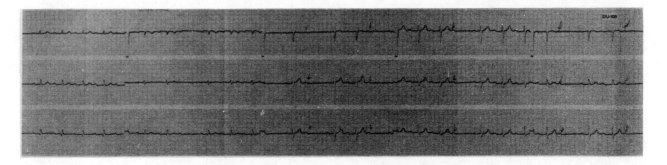

EKG 108

1. What does this record suggest?

ANSWER: Second-degree A-V block is present. The P-R interval ranges from .32 sec to .40 sec, to infinity, typical of Wenckebach phenomenon. This form of second-degree block is likely to be related to A-V nodal dysfunction and is often responsive to anticholinergic drugs. Often, it is self-limiting, unlike Mobitz II block, which is likely to be associated with constant bundle branch block, complicated by intermittent bilateral bundle branch block. These bundles lie below the region of vagal innervation, which does not extend into the ventricular myocardium; therefore, Mobitz II block seldom responds to anticholinergic drugs.

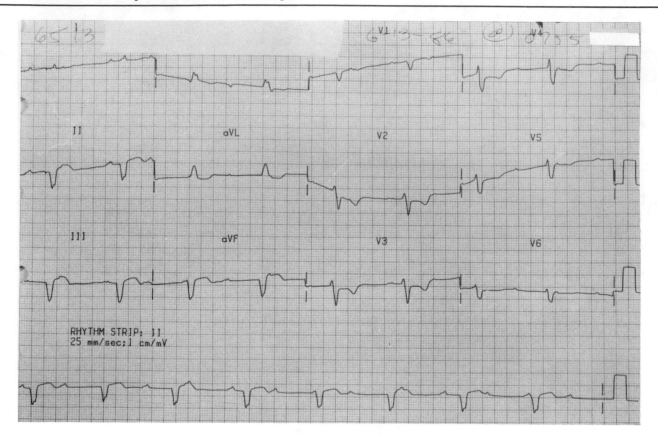

II   aVL   V2   V5

III   aVF   V3   V6

RHYTHM STRIP: II
25 mm/sec;1 cm/mV

EKG 109

1. Is this record a third-degree A-V block?

ANSWER: The constant R-R interval with varying *apparent* P-R interval indicates complete (third-degree) block. At times, high-grade second-degree block may resemble complete block. Regular R-R interval as noted here serves to distinguish second- from third-degree block.

2. Where is the ventricular pacemaker?

ANSWER: In wide QRS complexes with latest R waves in leads I and aVL, the final cells to lose their positive surface charges (last to depolarize) face the left shoulder and, therefore, are in the free wall of the left ventricle. Depolarization either originates in the right ventricle or advances into the ventricles over the right bundle (LBBB) from a focus in the AV junction or His bundle.

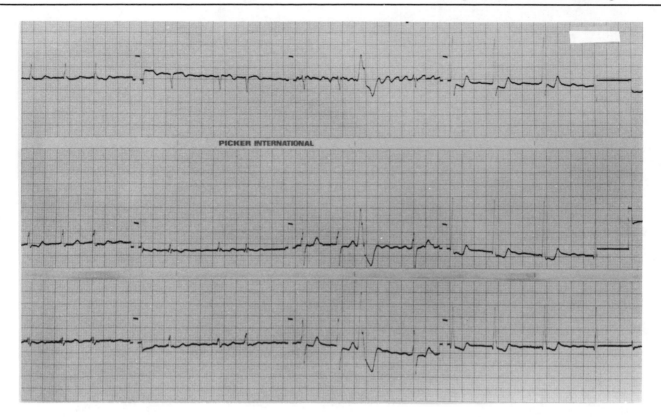

EKG 110

This record presents some information that is beyond debate and other features that can lead to useful speculation.

1. What would you propose?

ANSWER: The atrial fibrillation and ventricular premature contractions are diagnostic. The configuration of the ventricular premature contractions suggests that they originate in the posterior myocardium (possibly debatable).

The prominent atrial waves are considered by some to be compatible with atrial-wall hypertrophy, as in the presence of valvular disease (controversial). This patient does, in fact, have severe mitral regurgitation.

The S-T,T configuration is compatible with digitalis effect. Note that the voltage is not sufficient to be diagnostic of left ventricular hypertrophy. The patient is receiving digitalis. The echocardiographic data do *not* reveal left ventricular hypertrophy.

SELECTED READINGS

An encyclopedic bibliography is not my intention. The following reading selections include some that are of historic interest and others that relate to the basic concepts and clinical correlations fundamental to the presentation of this book.

1. Arvan, S., and Varat, M.A.: Persistent ST-segment elevation and left ventricular wall abnormalities: A 2-dimensional echocardiographic study. Am. J. Cardiol., *53:*1542, 1984.

2. Berne, R.M., and Levy, M.N.: Electrical activity of the heart. *In* Berne, R.M., and Levy, M.N.: Cardiovascular Physiology. St. Louis, C.V. Mosby, 1986.

3. Brunken, R., Tillisch, J., Schwaiger, M., et al.: Regional perfusion, glucose metabolism, and wall motion in patients with chronic electrocardiographic Q wave infarctions: Evidence for persistence of viable tissue in some infarct regions by positron emission tomography. Circulation, *73:*951, 1986.

4. Cranefield, P.F.: The Conduction of the Cardiac Impulse. Mt. Kisco, NY, Futura, 1975.

5. Cranefield, P.F., and Hoffman, B.: Electrophysiology of the Heart. New York, Mc-Graw-Hill, 1960.

6. Einthoven, W., Fahr, G., and de Waart, A.: Uber die Richtung und die manifeste grosse der Potentialschwankungen im menschlichen Herzen und uber Einfluss der Herzlage auf die Form des Elektrokardiogramms. Arch. f.d.g. Physiol., *150:*275, 1913.

7. Holland, R.P., and Brooks, H.: TQ-ST segment mapping: Critical review and analysis of current concepts. Am. J. Cardiol., *40:*110, 1977.

8. Horan, L.G., Hand, R.C., Johnson, J.C., et al.: A Theoretical examination of ventricular repolarization and the secondary T wave. Circ. Res., *42:*750, 1978.

9. Josephson, M.E., and Seides, S.F.: Clinical Cardiac Electrophysiology: Techniques and Interpretations. Philadelphia, Lea & Febiger, 1979.

10. Kannel, W.B., and Abbott, R.D.: A prognostic comparison of asymptomatic left ventricular hypertrophy and unrecognized myocardial infarction: the Framingham Study. Am. Heart J., *111:*391, 1986.

11. Lewis, T., Drury, A.N., and Iliescu, C.C.: A demonstration of circus movement in clinical flutter of the auricles. Heart, *8:*341, 1921.

12. Lewis, T., and Rothschild, M.A.: The excitatory process in the dog's heart: II. The ventricles. Trans. R. Soc. Lond. (B), *206:*181, 1915.

13. MacDonald, R.G., Hill, J.A., and Feldman, R.L.: ST segment response to acute coronary occlusion: Coronary hemodynamic and angiographic determinants of direction of ST segment shift. Circulation, *74:*973, 1986.

14. Mines, G.R.: On dynamic equilibrum in the heart. J. Physiol., *46:*349, 1913.

15. Montague, T.J., Johnstone, D.E., Spencer, C.A., et al.: Non-Q-wave acute myocardial infarction: Body surface potential map and ventriculographic patterns. Am. J. Cardiol., *58:*1173, 1986.

16. Murphy, M.L., Thenabadu, P.N., DeSoyza, N., et al.: Reevaluation of electrocardiographic criteria for left, right and combined cardiac ventricular hypertrophy. Am. J. Cardiol., *53:*1140, 1984.

17. Nademanee, K., Intarachot, V., Singh, P.N., et al.: Characteristics and clinical significance of silent myocardial ischemia in unstable angina. Am. J. Cardiol., *58:*26B, 1986.

18. Nesto, R.W., and Phillips, R.T.: Silent myocardial ischemia: Clinical characteristics, underlying mechanisms, and implications for treatment. Am. J. Med., *81:*12, 1986.

19. Nobel, D.: The initiation of the heartbeat. Oxford, Clarendon Press, 1975.

20. Odom, H., Davis, J.L., Dinh, H., et al.: QRS voltage measurements in autopsied men free of cardiopulmonary disease: A basis for evaluating total QRS voltage as an index of left ventricular hypertrophy. Am. J. Cardiol., *58:*801, 1986.

21. Reuter, H.: Ion channels in cardiac cell membranes. Ann. Rev. Physiol., *46:*473, 1984.

22. Rosenbaum, M.B., Elizari, M.V., and Lazzari, J.O.: The Hemiblocks. Oldsmar, FL, Tampa Tracings, 1970.

23. Ruddy, T.D., Yasuda, T., Gold, H.K., et al.: Anterior ST-segment depression in acute in-

ferior myocardial infarction as a marker of greater inferior, apical, and posterolateral damage. Am. Heart J., *112:*1210, 1986.

24. Schamroth, L.: The Electrocardiology of Coronary Artery Disease. London, Blackwell Scientific Publications, 1975.

25. Scharovsky, S., Davidson, E., Lewin, R.F., et al.: Unstable angina pectoris evolving to acute myocardial infarction: Significance of ECG changes during chest pain. Am. Heart J., *112:*459, 1986.

26. Scharovsky, S., Davidson, E., Strasberg, B., et al.: Unstable angina: The significance of ST segment elevation or depression in patients without evidence of increased myocardial oxygen demand. Am. Heart J., *112:*463, 1986.

27. Schwartz, P.J., and Wolf, S.: QT interval prolongation as predictor of sudden death in patients with myocardial infarction. Circulation, *57:*1074, 1978.

28. Van Dam, R.T., and Durrer, D.: The T wave and ventricular repolarization. Am. J. Cardiol., *14:*294, 1964.

29. Wallace, A.G., Sealy, W.C., Gallagher, J.J. and Kasell, J.: Ventricular excitation in Wolff-Parkinson-White syndrome. *In* H.J.J. Wellens, K.I. Lie, and M.J. Janse (eds.): The Conduction System of the Heart: Structure, Function and Clinical Implications. Leiden, H.E. Stenfert Kroese BV, 1976.

30. Wellens, H.J.: Bishop Lecture: The electrocardiogram 80 years after Einthoven (Review). Am. Coll. Cardiol., *7:*484, 1986.

31. Wilson, F.N.: Foreword. *In* Barker, J.M.: The Unipolar Electrogram: A Clinical Interpretation. New York, Appleton-Century-Crofts, 1952.

32. Woythaler, J.N., Singer, S.L., Kwan, O.L., et al.: Accuracy of echocardiography versus electrocardiography in detecting left ventricular hypertrophy: Comparison with postmortem mass measurements. J. Am. Coll. Cardiol., *2:*305, 1983.

APPENDIX:

Computer Generation
of the
Electrocardiogram

Recognizing the relationship between single-cell electrical phenomena and the electrocardiogram as presented in the first section of this book, one of us (D.M.D.) conceived of a means of evaluating these associations by computer modeling of the myocardium. He arranged 350 to 400 representative "cells" in horizontal and frontal plane maps of the ventricles. Each normal cell was assigned a 90-mV resting potential. "Cells" were depolarized in normal sequence, and their action potentials were given normal configurations and durations with surface charge represented at 10-msec intervals. The computer, as directed by Dye's program, scans the model and identifies the areas where there are cells near one another with significantly different potentials. Thus, the computer recognizes the wave fronts of depolarization and repolarization. The computer averages the charges found on these cells, recognizes that array of cells whose charges are more positive and more negative than this average, and resolves these areas of positive and negative charge into a dipole. The dipole vectors are projected on the 12 conventional electrocardiographic leads so as to derive the electrocardiogram.

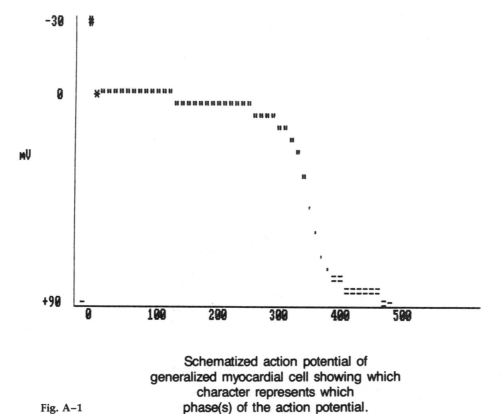

Fig. A–1

Schematized action potential of
generalized myocardial cell showing which
character represents which
phase(s) of the action potential.

Figure A–1 demonstrates the charge symbols of a normal action potential in the presence of 90-mV resting potential.

Figure A–2a–k presents a series of horizontal plane maps of the left ventricle. The symbols indicate charges as depicted in Figure A–1.

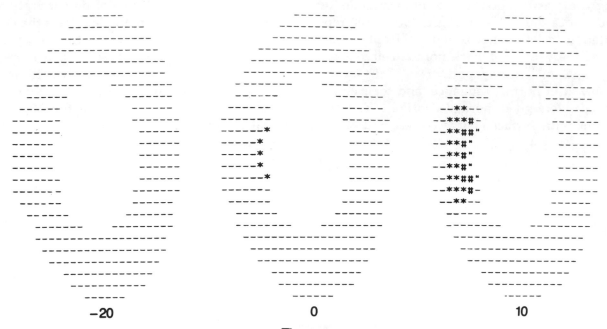

Time: msec

a

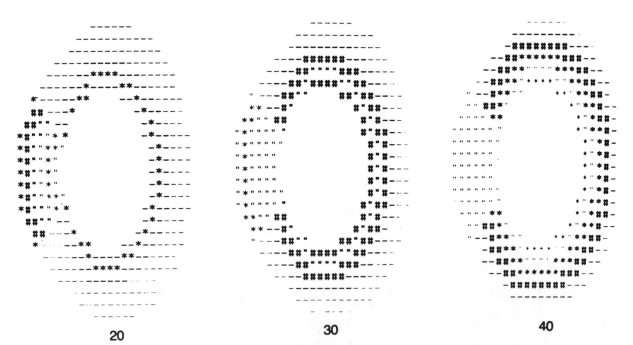

Time: msec

b

Fig. A–2

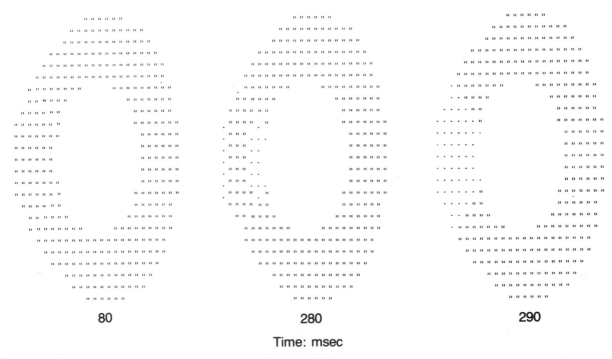

Fig. A–2 Continued.

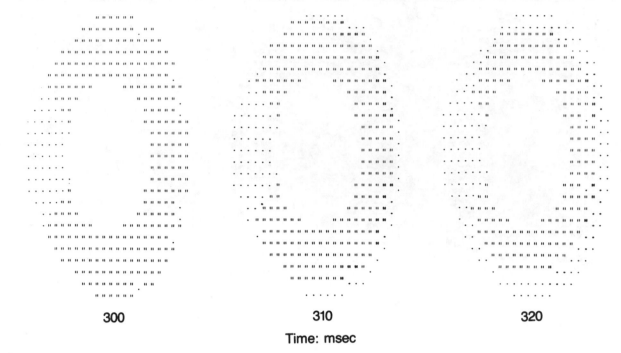

300   310   320

Time: msec

e

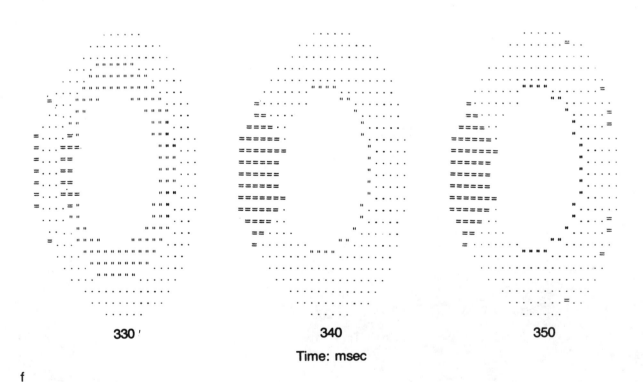

330   340   350

Time: msec

f

Fig. A–2 Continued.

360 370 380

Time: msec

g

390 400 410

Time: msec

h

Fig. A–2 Continued.

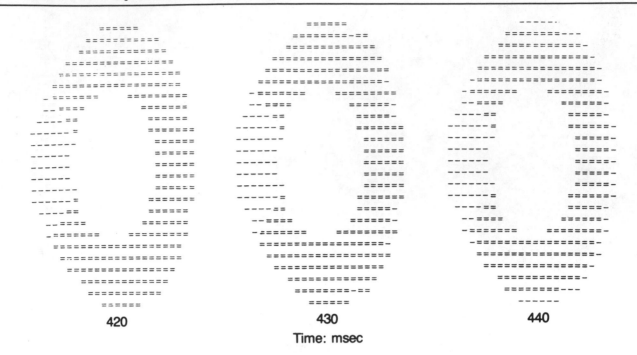

420   430   440

Time: msec

i

450   460   470

Time: msec

j

Fig. A–2 Continued.

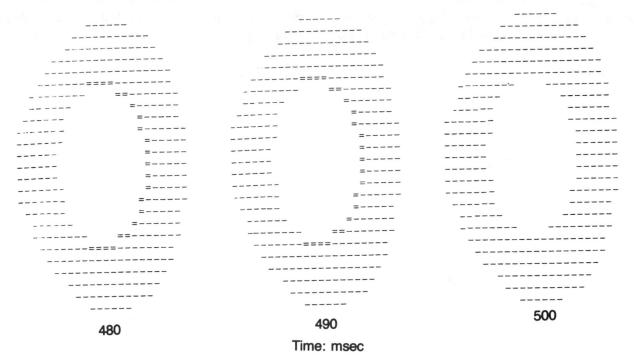

480   490   500
                  Time: msec

k

Fig. A–2 Continued.

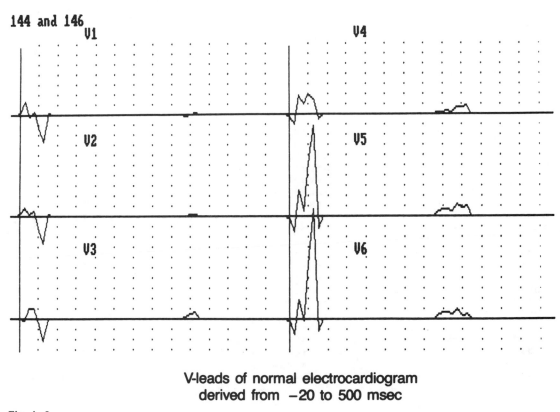

144 and 146

V-leads of normal electrocardiogram
derived from −20 to 500 msec

Fig. A–3

Figure A–3 presents the derived V leads of this
normal model.

Figure A–4a–1 is the frontal plane map of the normal left ventricular depolarization and repolarization. From 100 msec to 290 msec all cells are depolarized and no change takes place (e).

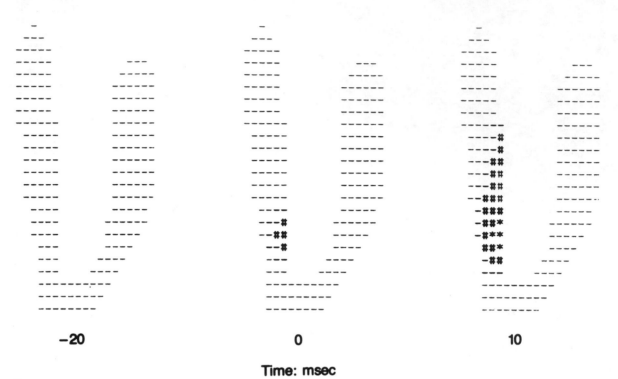

a

b

Fig. A–4

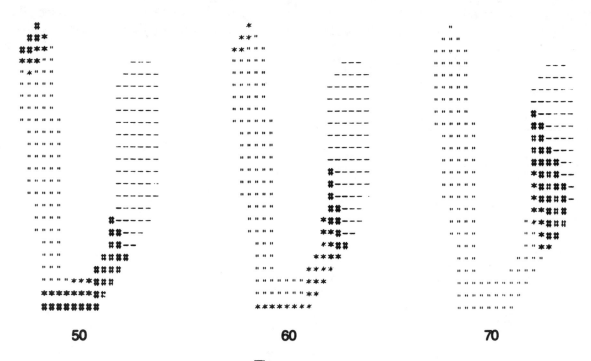

50   60   70

Time: msec

c

80   90   100

Time: msec

d

Fig. A–4 Continued.

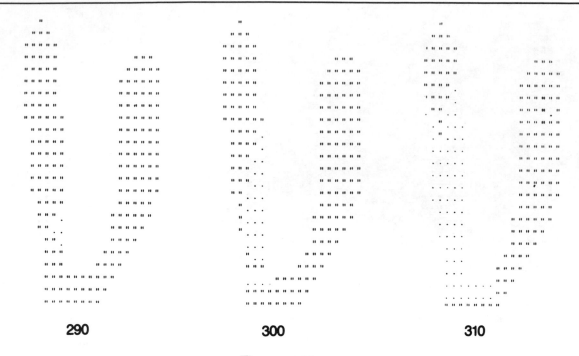

290　　　　　　**300**　　　　　　**310**

Time: msec

e

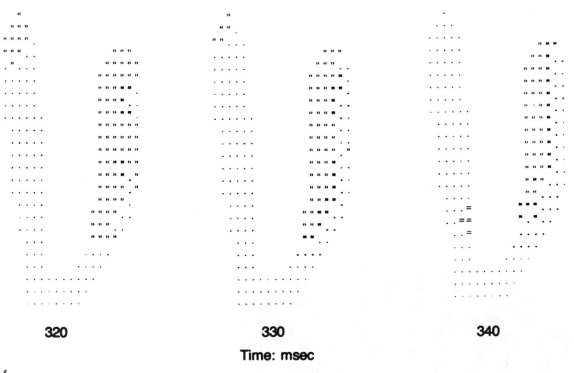

320　　　　　　**330**　　　　　　**340**

Time: msec

f

Fig. A–4 Continued.

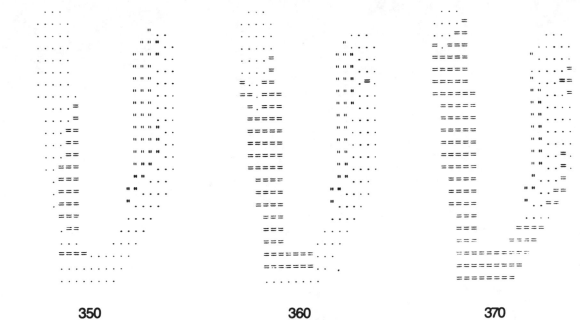

350   360   370

Time: msec

g

380   390   400

Time: msec

h

Fig. A–4 Continued.

410   420   430

Time: msec

i

440   450   460

Time: msec

j

Fig. A–4 Continued.

470   480   490

Time: msec

k

500   510   520   530

Time: msec

l

Fig. A–4 Continued.

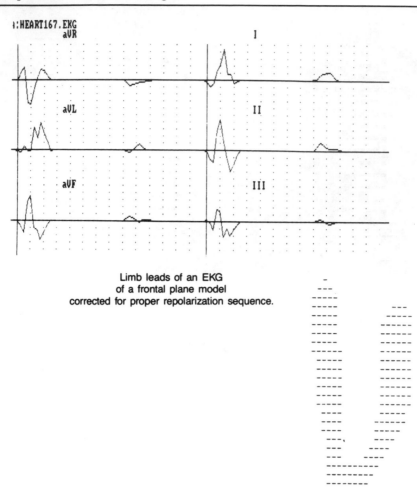

Fig. A–5

Figure A–5 shows derived frontal plane leads.

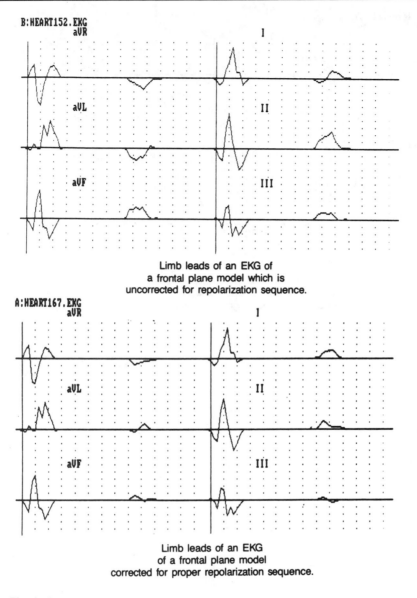

Limb leads of an EKG of
a frontal plane model which is
uncorrected for repolarization sequence.

Limb leads of an EKG
of a frontal plane model
corrected for proper repolarization sequence.

Fig. A–6

Figure A–6 illustrates the effect of a slight
change in angular repolarization of the free wall
on the T waves, especially in aVL and aVF.

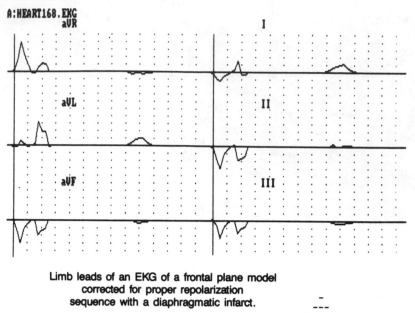

A:HEART168.EKG

Limb leads of an EKG of a frontal plane model
corrected for proper repolarization
sequence with a diaphragmatic infarct.

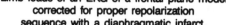

−20 msec

Fig. A–7

Figure A–7 shows a diaphragmatic myocardial
infarction.

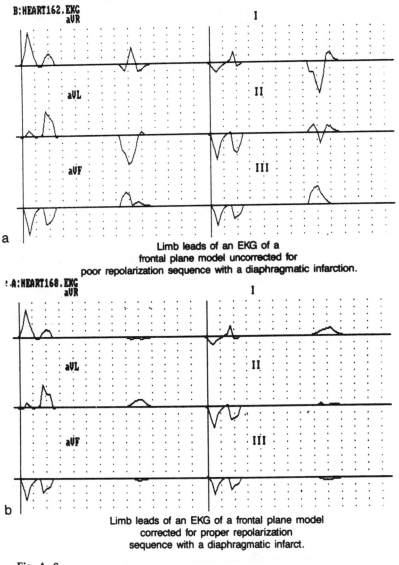

Limb leads of an EKG of a
frontal plane model uncorrected for
poor repolarization sequence with a diaphragmatic infarction.

Limb leads of an EKG of a frontal plane model
corrected for proper repolarization
sequence with a diaphragmatic infarct.

Fig. A–8

Figure A–8 shows the limb leads of an EKG in the presence of diaphragmatic infarction with anterolateral subendocardial ischemia (a); the same diaphragmatic infarction without anterolateral ischemia (b).

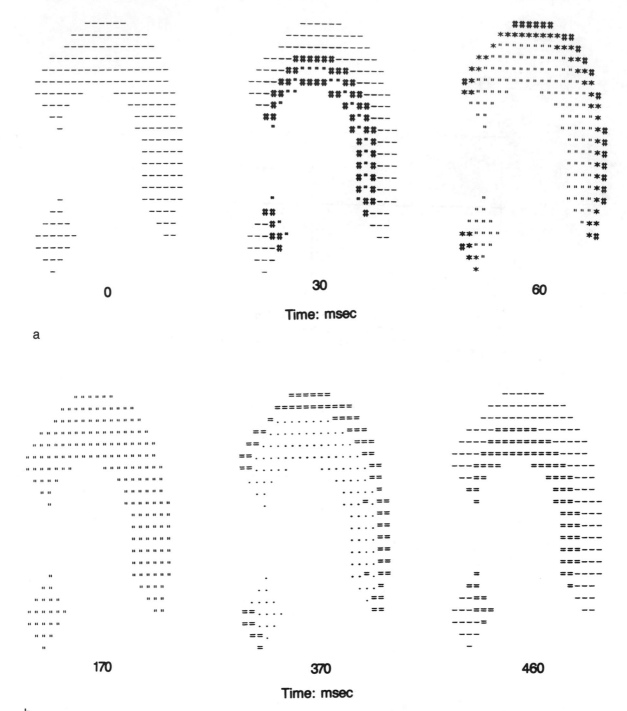

Fig. A–9

Figure A–9a and b presents anterolateral infarction maps of depolarization and repolarization with events recorded at 0, 30, 60, 170, 370, and 460 msec after the onset of phase 0. Please note that the interventricular septal segment has been omitted from this map.

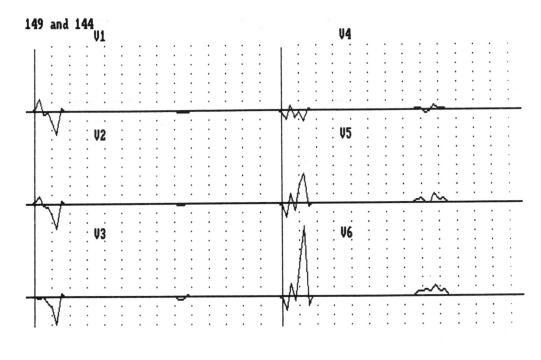

149 and 144

V-leads of electrocardiogram
derived in process of
anterolateral transmural infarct

Fig. A–10

The derived EKG is shown in Figure A–10.

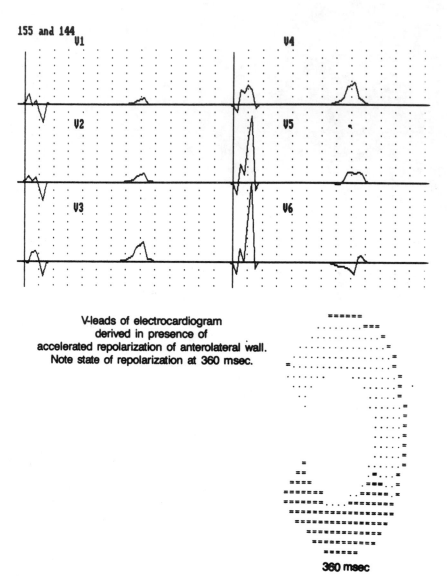

155 and 144

V-leads of electrocardiogram
derived in presence of
accelerated repolarization of anterolateral wall.
Note state of repolarization at 360 msec.

360 msec

Fig. A-11

Because ischemic cell damage may shorten or prolong the action potential, the computer has been directed to model these situations. Figure A-11 presents the map and the EKG in the presence of pathologic shortening of the action potential in an anterolateral region.

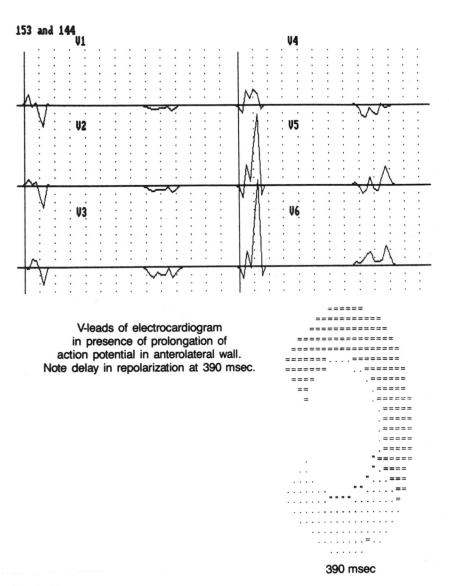

V-leads of electrocardiogram
in presence of prolongation of
action potential in anterolateral wall.
Note delay in repolarization at 390 msec.

390 msec

Fig. A–12

Figure A–12 demonstrates the effects of action
potential prolongation in this area.

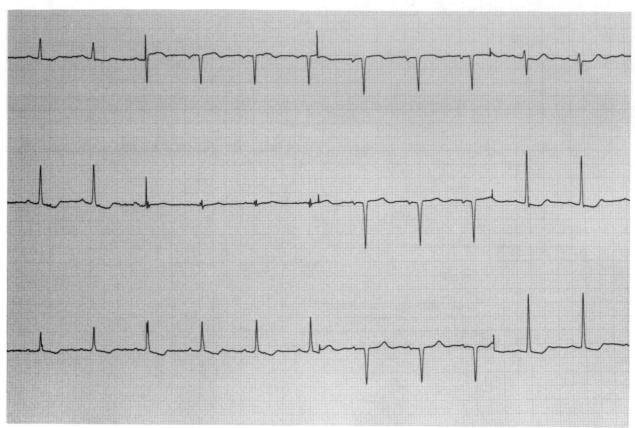

Fig. A–13

Figure A–13 is a clinical tracing of an antero-septal infarction. Note the upright T waves in leads V_2 and V_3 in the presence of QS in these leads. One explanation for the upright T in these leads is suggested by Figure A–11. If the surviving cells in the matrix of the infarct repolarize prematurely (short action potential), the effect would be to generate early positive charges directed at leads V_2 and V_3 during repolarization.

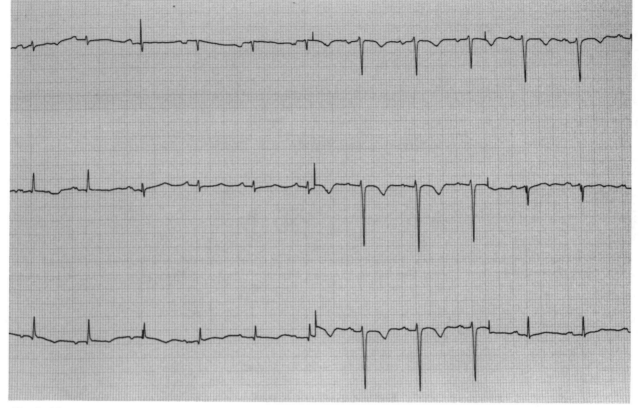

Fig. A–14

In Figure A–14 there are deep T inversions in the V leads in the presence of anteroseptal, anterior, and lateral ischemic damage, which almost certainly includes an anterolateral infarction. This T inversion may reflect (a) loss of cells; (b) pathologic prolongation of that action potential of sur-viving cells, with tardy generation of positivity directed anteriorly (overbalanced by the on-time repolarization of the opposite healthy wall); or (c) premature repolarization of the ischemic area, with greatest prematurity in the subendocardial area in which ischemic insult is greatest.

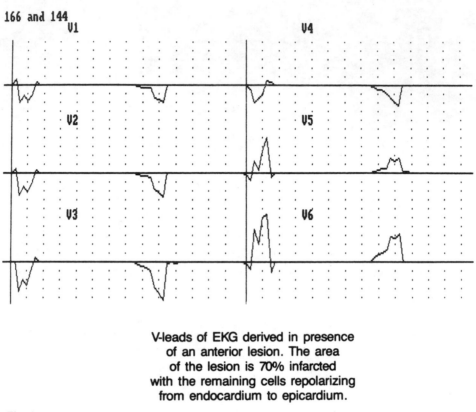

V-leads of EKG derived in presence
of an anterior lesion. The area
of the lesion is 70% infarcted
with the remaining cells repolarizing
from endocardium to epicardium.

Fig. A–15

Figure A–15 illustrates the computer model of this situation, in which, because action potential duration decreases progressively from epicardium to endocardium as in ischemia, a repolarizing dipole advances from endo- to epicardium with the negative leading edge directed at leads V_1 to V_4.

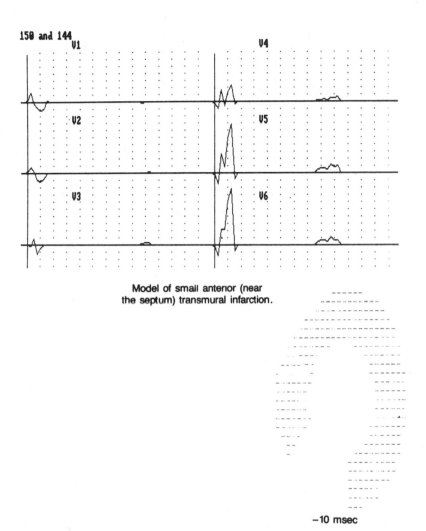

Model of small anterior (near
the septum) transmural infarction.

−10 msec

Fig. A–16

Figure A–16 illustrates the sensitivity of the computer model. Note the subtle loss of the .03-sec R wave in the anteroseptal leads in the presence of a small anteroseptal, anterior, and myocardial loss (compare with the normal V leads in Figure A–3).

Heart 171 LBBB

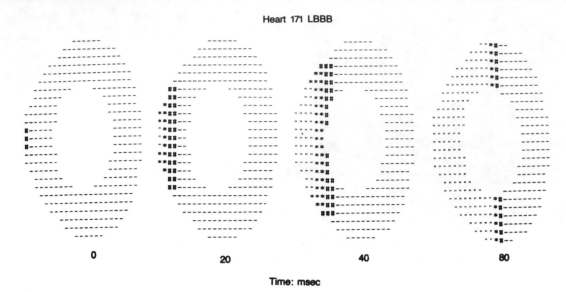

0   20   40   80

Time: msec

a

Heart 171 LBBB

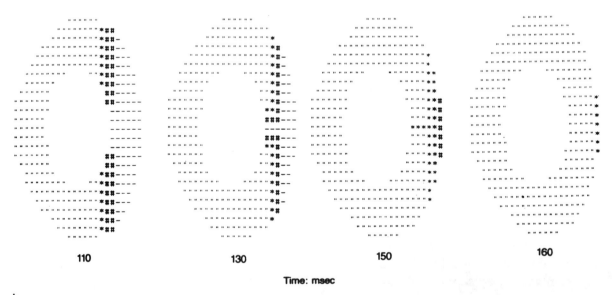

110   130   150   160

Time: msec

b

Fig. A–17

Left bundle branch block is shown in Figure
A–17a and b.

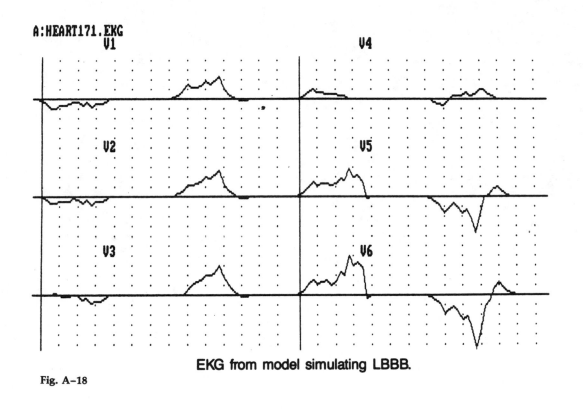

A:HEART171.EKG

EKG from model simulating LBBB.

Fig. A–18

The derived EKG is shown in Figure A–18.

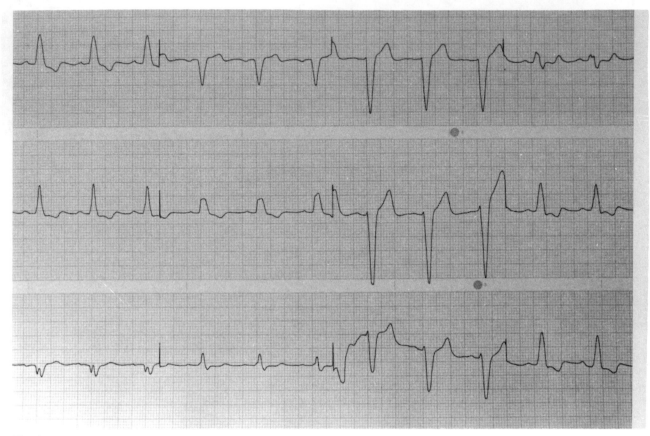

Fig. A–19

A clinical tracing with left bundle branch block
serves as a comparison (Figure A–19).

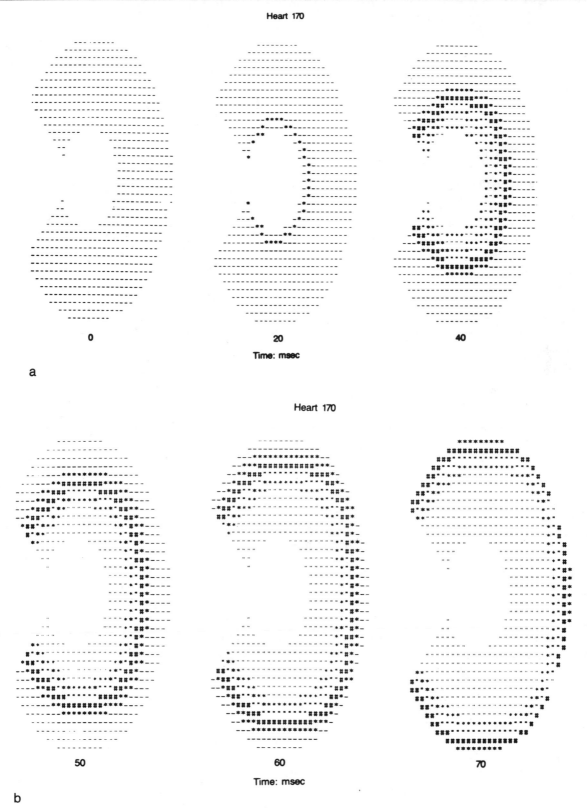

Heart 170

Time: msec

a

Heart 170

Time: msec

b

Fig. A–20

Figure A–20a and b presents the maps of left ventricular hypertrophy (LVH) in which a focal conduction delay occurs in the anteroseptal and posteroseptal areas (eight and ten o'clock).

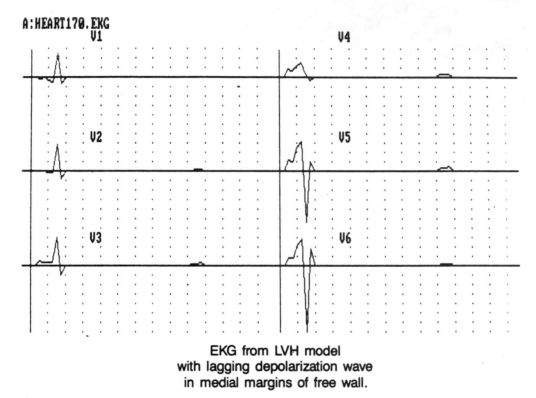

A:HEART170.EKG

EKG from LVH model
with lagging depolarization wave
in medial margins of free wall.

Fig. A–21

The derived EKG (Figure A–21) demonstrates the significant alterations that result. (Note the difference from LVH without conduction delay in Figure A–24).

Heart 176 LVE

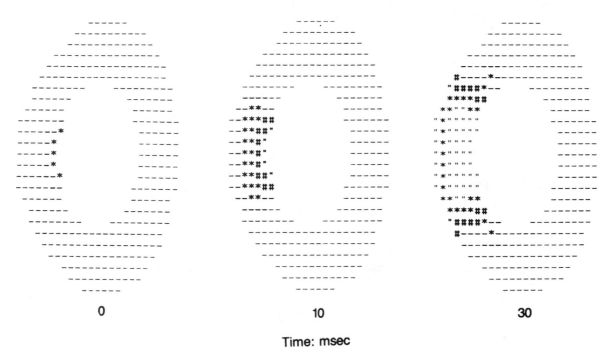

Time: msec

a

Heart 176 LVE

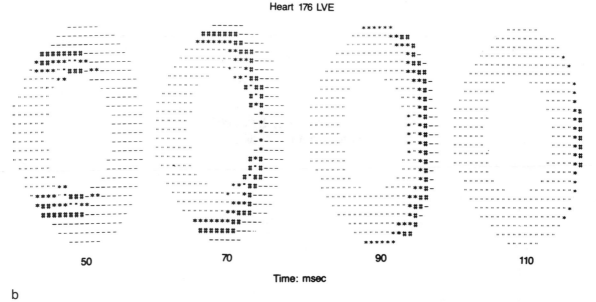

Time: msec

b

Fig. A–22

The effects of left ventricular dilatation are shown in Figure A–22a and b, and the modeled EKG is presented in Figure A–23. The conduction delay and modest increase in QRS voltage should be noted.

A:HEART176.EKG

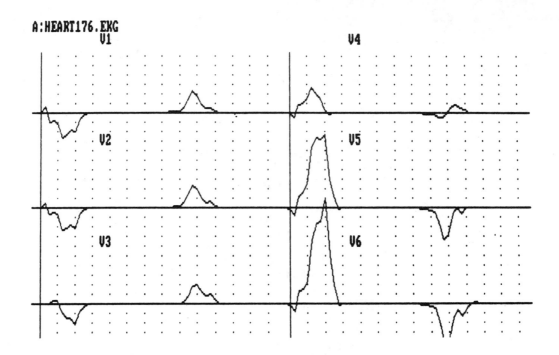

EKG generated by model
of left ventricular dilation.

Fig. A-23

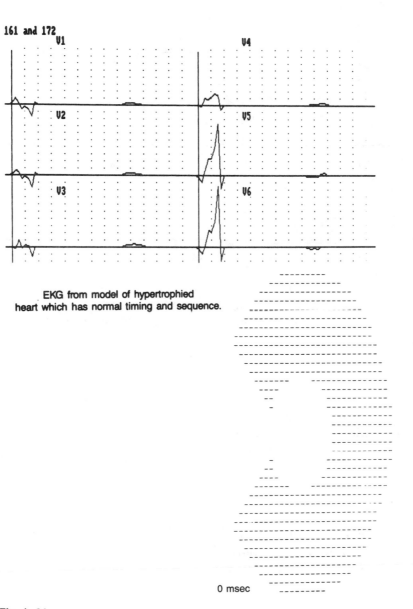

EKG from model of hypertrophied
heart which has normal timing and sequence.

0 msec

Fig. A-24

Figure A-24 represents increased left ventricular *mass* without *conduction delay*. Note the increased voltage and normal QRS duration and the retention of normal septal Q waves.

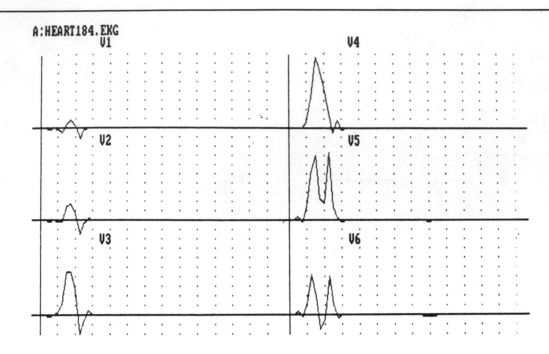

A:HEART184.EKG

**EKG generated by a model
which simulates left ventricular hypertrophy.**

Fig. A–25

Figure A–25 presents left ventricular hypertrophy with marked conduction delay and T-wave abnormalities.

A word should be added regarding the right ventricle in these models. Because the normal right ventricle makes no net contribution to the EKG, these models without right ventricular disease have been presented without a right ventricular component.

Index

Page numbers in *italics* indicate figures.